W9-BQU-538

Yoga

for WOMEN at MIDLIFE & BEYOND

A H O M E C O M P A N I O N

Yoga

for WOMEN at MIDLIFE & BEYOND

A HOME COMPANION

Pat Shapiro, MSW, RYT

Illustrations by Jaye Oliver
Photographs by Thea Witt

SUNSTONE PRESS

SANTA FE

Illustrations by Jaye Oliver
Photographs by Thea Witt
Book and cover design by Vicki Ahl

© 2006 by Pat Shapiro. All rights reserved.

No part of this book may be reproduced in any form or by any electronic or mechanical means including information storage and retrieval systems without permission in writing from the publisher, except by a reviewer who may quote brief passages in a review.

Sunstone books may be purchased for educational, business, or sales promotional use. For information please write: Special Markets Department, Sunstone Press, P.O. Box 2321, Santa Fe, New Mexico 87504-2321.

Library of Congress Cataloging-in-Publication Data:

Shapiro, Patricia Gottlieb.
 Yoga for women at midlife & beyond : a home companion / by Pat Shapiro ; illustrations by Jaye Oliver ; photographs by Thea Witt.
    p. cm.
  ISBN 0-86534-499-X (softcover : alk. paper)
 1. Hatha yoga. 2. Middle-aged persons--Health and hygiene. 3. Older people--Health and hygiene. I. Title. II. Title: Yoga for women at midlife and beyond.

RA781.7.S4385 2006
613.7'0460844--dc22

                                         2006023427

Published in

WWW.SUNSTONEPRESS.COM
SUNSTONE PRESS / POST OFFICE BOX 2321 / SANTA FE, NM 87504-2321 /USA
(505) 988-4418 / ORDERS ONLY (800) 243-5644 / FAX (505) 988-1025

To my teacher
Sonia Nelson
for her wisdom and support
and
for my students
who have taught me
patience and compassion

Contents

Foreword

I've practiced and taught yoga for the past thirty years and if I had to use one word to express the way it has influenced me, what immediately comes to mind is "support." In her book, Pat Shapiro shows how in every area of life the practice of yoga can be an adaptable tool that supports intentions and interactions on a day-to-day basis. From the purely physical to the deeply spiritual, from the energetic to the intellectual to the psychological, yoga practice supports our attempts to remain physically healthy, increase and conserve energy, refine and manifest intellectual potential, transform confusion into clarity, and heal the inevitable aches and pains of the heart as well as the body.

Pat not only provides the techniques that make yoga practice effective, but she has provided the extra element of care and support that is often missing from instructional material. Trying to establish a regular home yoga practice can be challenging in many ways and the support Pat offers throughout this book will go a long way in helping you transform the idea of yoga practice into a reality.

—Sonia Nelson
Santa Fe, New Mexico

A Note to the Reader:

The information in this book is for educational purposes only. It is not intended as medical advice or to replace the guidance of a physician or health care professional. Please consult your health care provider before beginning this or any exercise program. The author and publisher accept no responsibility or liability for injuries that may have resulted from use of the information in this book.

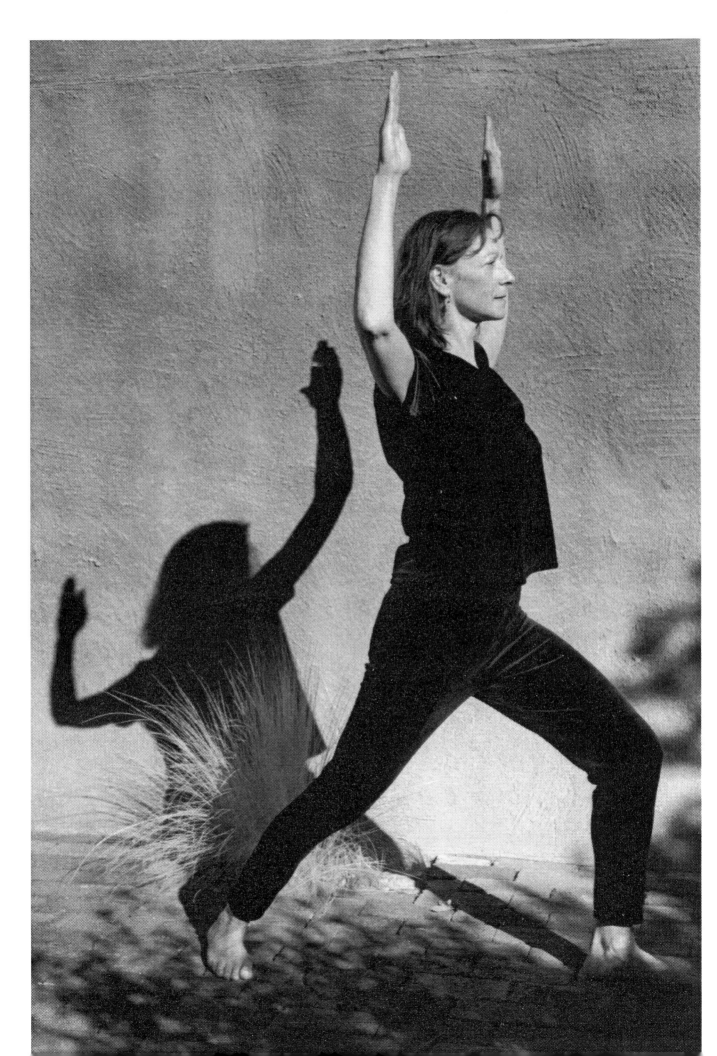

1

Yoga at Midlife

Yoga is a homecoming, a coming home—to ourselves.

We all want that, no matter what our age. For most of us at midlife and older, our parents have passed on or are in a frail condition; they are not the same people we grew up with. We can no longer return to the childhood home where we grew up. But we can recreate—internally—the feelings of safety, comfort and contentment that we experienced. If you didn't experience these feelings growing up, you can recapture those times later in your life when you did feel safe. Perhaps you felt this way nursing your first child, or feel it lying on the beach, or hiking in the woods.

The first time I did yoga, I walked into a small studio bathed in white. Something about the atmosphere made me feel relaxed and calm—even before I did any postures. It was a difficult time in my life. I needed peace and a respite from a set of family problems. I walked in feeling uptight and edgy. When I walked out after class, I was in another place. The problems were still there but they didn't seem as bad. They felt more distant. And I was less emotional about them.

When I do yoga I feel as though I've come home. It doesn't matter where I do it. I am home.

Yoga helps us feel comfortable in our own skin. We're past the age of trying to impress others. We don't need to conform to be part of a group. We just want to be ourselves, and act and respond out of our own authenticity.

Yoga means union, or to unite or come together. We can interpret that in many ways. Some believe it means union with God or a higher power. Others say yoga occurs when our attention is directed only toward the activity we are engaged in.

For me, the union or the wholeness is internal: feeling at one with myself. When I feel this way, I'm better able to meet the crises and challenges that are a natural part of living. I can handle difficult situations with more confidence, because I am connected to my inner voice and respond from my core, rather than being unduly influenced by those around me. My practice keeps me centered and steady.

You may think that by the time you're 50, you're already at peace with yourself. But that's not necessarily so. Many of us have conflicts and regrets at this age. We think, I would have, could have, should have done this or that. Some of us have issues from childhood that have never been resolved.

And then things happen that throw you off kilter: your best friend moves across the country, a child or grandchild gets sick, your marriage dissolves. These situations would challenge anyone. But when you're doing yoga regularly, you're able to meet situations like these with more composure and poise. You recover faster and lose your equilibrium less easily and less often.

"At age thirteen, I had the good fortune of being introduced to yoga when my school offered it as a physical education elective. I loved learning about the body-mind-heart connection and found myself using the poses and breath work outside of class to help me cope with the emotional turmoil of adolescence. Yoga classes continued to be a part of my life in college, but when I married, started a family, and pursued a career, my practice of yoga drifted away.

"Now at mid-life, yoga has called to me again. In this time of hormonal and life changes, I need the calming, stretching, and breathing of yoga to stay healthy, flexible, and balanced. Practicing yoga keeps my energy open and flowing, and helps me nourish the vitality that might otherwise wane with age.

"Looking back, I realize that even when I was not actively practicing yoga, the early training of body-mind-heart connection continued to influence my cultivation of a balanced, aware, and compassionate life. Yoga will now be a life-long practice for me; the benefits are truly timeless!"

—Naomi C. Rose, 50 (shown on page 12)

What is Yoga?

Yoga is difficult to define because it encompasses so many aspects of living and being, and means so many different things to different people. In the west, people tend to define yoga as a form of exercise and think of it as set of postures and movements. In Sanskrit this is called *asana*. In truth, this is one part of yoga, obviously the most well-known part. Yoga also includes the practice of conscious breathing, tools to bring about a meditative state of mind, as well as many principles for living, such as our attitudes to ourselves and to others.

Yoga is a philosophy, a way of life, and a spiritual practice. It is not connected with any particular religion and does not require a specific belief system. If you have your own belief system or religious conviction, the practice of yoga will not challenge it.

Because of the way the origin of yoga has been portrayed, some people think "a yogi" is someone who lives alone on a mountaintop, meditating for 12 hours a day, divorced from civilization. This may have been true in the past, but that scenario is no longer relevant. We live in the real world. We have homes, families, jobs, and friends. Yoga offers useful lessons in how to live our lives.

Yoga is about action. It's about setting an intention, following through, and being attentive to our behavior and to our relationships. It's about observing and acknowledging the obstacles that keep us from acting decisively and consciously, and taking the steps to face and overcome them.

Originating in India approximately 3000 years ago, yoga was passed on through generations as an oral tradition. Today, we have a whole body of written works expounding and interpreting the philosophy for modern times and documenting its effectiveness as a tool for enhancing our lives in the midst of this complex twenty-first century. Yoga has survived for hundreds of years because the principles are ageless and timeless. They are just as pertinent today as they were centuries ago.

Your Practice is Not Your Daughter's Practice

The latest trend is that yoga is for everybody and for every body. I believe this as much as the next person, but that doesn't mean that a practice that's right for a 25-year-old woman is also appropriate for someone who is 50 years old. Women at midlife and older have special needs, just as women who are pregnant have particular needs. It is possible to develop a practice for each specialized group that is appropriate for their unique situation.

This means we need to modify our practices to acknowledge our age and the stage of life we are in. We live in such a youth-oriented culture (epitomized by all the svelte young bodies on the covers of yoga magazines) that it's easy to be influenced by these images. Making that image a goal, however, may not be the best thing for our health or wellbeing.

The emphasis of practice changes, as we get older. At 30 you may have thrilled at accomplishing a handstand or doing 12 Sun Salutations without stopping. At midlife, we still need stretching and strengthening, but we're more interested in protecting and preserving our physical and emotional health than in perfecting postures. This means that if we wake up with stiffness, we may need to do more warm ups. Or we may do fewer poses or choose to concentrate on simpler ones, or we may decide to practice in a chair because we're low on energy or need external support to help stabilize us.

We also become more reflective as we reach midlife. We've experienced loss on many levels and we've weathered experiences that have made us stronger and have increased our compassion for others and for ourselves.

With the awareness that midlife brings comes a yearning for a more meaningful life. We want to stay fit and limber but many of us also come to yoga searching for something deeper: a stronger link to our inner voice, a way to understand our place in the changing world, and a more relevant spiritual connection.

Consequently, we become more interested in the

meditative aspects and rewards of yoga. A practice that is purely physical is less satisfying as we get older. We're drawn to the multi-layered meaning of yoga and its implications for our lives. This may result in a shorter *asana* practice and a longer meditation; or doing a leisurely, meditative practice focusing on the breath, rather than a physically demanding one; and setting aside time to study and contemplate ideas from classical yoga philosophy.

Whatever form your practice takes, you will reap benefits. Your strength, energy and flexibility will increase. Your balance will improve. You'll sleep better and feel sharper mentally. You'll begin to develop an inner sense of calm that will enable you to meet challenging situations with self-assurance and certainty.

Most importantly, yoga can help you age with grace and vitality. Yoga encourages self-reflection and teaches us awareness, acceptance and gratitude. Through yoga, we learn to live in the moment and cherish each day.

Why This Approach Works Well for Older Women

There are many different styles, approaches and traditions of yoga. You need to find the one that resonates with you. Practically speaking, you might consider the approach of the studios in your neighborhood, so you can support your personal practice by attending classes.

I study an approach to yoga that was brought to the West through the teaching of T.K.V. Desikachar and his students. T.K.V. Desikachar was the closest student of his father, Professor Tirumalai Krishnamacharya, who taught and influenced many prominent teachers in the West, including Pattabhi Jois, B.K.S. Iyengar and Indra Devi.

One of the benchmarks of this approach is that the postures are adapted to fit the needs of the individual. So, rather than asking *you* to conform to an ideal or perfect posture, this approach encourages you to let the posture conform to *your* needs. This means that each posture is tailored to your particular body type and size, to your flexibility, and to your strengths and weaknesses. This is particularly relevant as we get older, because many of us no longer have thin, toned bodies and have developed physical or structural problems, as we've gotten older. Keeping the intention of the posture, we can add variations that are appropriate for our bodies and our particular conditions.

This approach also emphasizes that function is more important than form—another relevant concept at midlife. Again, we use the classical posture as an ideal but modify it as we learn about ourselves *while we are in the postures*. We do the postures from the inside out. As we practice, we can ask ourselves: How does this posture feel on the inside? How is my body responding to the movement or to holding this posture? We observe ourselves in practice and then can make modifications as needed.

In this approach, we also do the postures dynamically before we hold them. That means we go in and out of the posture before we stay. And we don't always stay in a posture, particularly if we are new to yoga. If a posture is new to you, it's better to do it dynamically until you gain a sense of what is required to stay. When you're ready to stay, do it in gradual increments, measured by the number of breaths you feel comfortable with in that particular posture.

Finally, in this approach, there is a strong emphasis on the breath. Throughout our entire practice, the breath guides us and is the key to our state of mind. In everyday living our breathing is unconscious; it happens whether or not we think about it. In yoga practice, we consciously slow down and coordinate our breathing with our movement, making the movement last as long as the breath.

We'll talk more about the specific uses of the breath in Chapter 3, but for now keep in mind that by influencing the nature and quality of the breath, we bring a new attentiveness to our practice, and our chattering minds become more restrained. Once we master this, we can bring this remarkable quality into our daily lives.

"My practice of yoga began after I turned fifty, a somewhat literal midlife event, and one which marked an abrupt shift in what I knew of life, that is marriage and a large family. At a friend's suggestion, I attended a weekly yoga class and began to shape a home practice that, over the years, included asana, meditation and journaling.

"From the present perspective of eighteen years, yoga has given me a unique ability to bring together—to yoke—and to give a daily focus, to discipline, and to measure shifts in the body, in emotional stability, in mental ease. This has been my experience of recent years in creating a practice at home under the guidance of a teacher. With her, I am able to allow a natural pace to evolve, not straining, not setting goals, staying quite simply with what is happening now in this breath, this posture, this gesture or chant. The whole organism has a chance to catch up, to center, to concentrate. There is room then for whatever happens or not, and for me, to quite simply, be present.

"Yoga has been the thread, beginning early in the process and now, has become the focus. I have simplified my daily life, with few claims on time or energy. I am very grateful this is possible."

—Ellen Taylor, 68

Yoga and You

We all know that yoga is not an exercise like biking or running. But because yoga does involve movement, people tend to bring their attitudes toward sports to their practice. These attitudes can be detrimental, because they interfere with one of the goals of yoga, which is to be nonjudgmental and accepting of ourselves.

Yoga is completely noncompetitive. It doesn't matter that the person next to you in class can balance on one foot longer than you can, or that her form looks better in a particular pose. Each of you is a different individual with a different body, a different history, and a different mindset. You each have your own strengths and limitations. And you are each in a different place every single day.

In yoga practice, we even avoid competing with ourselves. Perhaps you were able to hold a posture longer yesterday than today. Rather than criticizing yourself or pushing yourself unnecessarily, we learn to accept that this is where we are at this point in time. There may be a very good reason for the difference: maybe you didn't sleep well last night or your mind is preoccupied because of distressing news you received before you began practicing. All these things have an impact.

It helps to keep in mind one of the concepts from classic yoga philosophy: the idea that everything changes. One day you can balance on one foot for a full minute; the next day you can't even stand for a few seconds. Or, your allergies are terrible today. You can't go out of the house without having a sneezing fit. You feel like the allergy season will never end. Yoga philosophy tells us that what you're experiencing is real but it will change. We'll discuss this in more depth later, but simply knowing this can give you a broader perspective on your varying responses to your practice.

In doing sports, you may experience pain and force yourself to push through the pain and keep going, no matter what the consequence. In yoga, if you feel pain, find a variation of the posture that doesn't hurt or stop what you're doing altogether. If you're in a class, tell the teacher. If you're practicing at home and don't know a variation, end the posture and rest. There's one exception: If you're inexperienced in stretching and are not that flexible, you may feel some muscle soreness from the newness of the posture. This is different. This is not pain but a good kind of discomfort that shows that you're expanding in new ways.

About This Book

Yoga for Women at Midlife & Beyond: A Home Companion is a manual for any woman over 50 who needs guidance about how to start a personal practice in the privacy of her own home. It is for women who are currently enrolled in yoga classes as well as for those who prefer to practice on their own.

This book contains guidelines on how to create a home practice that works with the space you have available and with your lifestyle. I'll give examples of how other women have used an area in their home to design a sacred space in an imaginative way, and include ideas for transforming an office and carving out a corner in your bedroom.

The book also devotes a chapter to the mechanics of yoga breathing with suggestions for integrating breath and movement during yoga practice. Another chapter includes ten practices with illustrations that you can follow on your own, such as a practice for energy, one for relaxation and another for insomnia. There is also information on how to begin a meditation practice at home. In addition, the book introduces concepts from classical yoga philosophy and raises questions to help you think about integrating these concepts into your life. Scattered throughout the book are stories from women at midlife and older that reveal how yoga has made a difference in their lives.

Getting Started

Begin where you are. You are reading this book, so you're probably interested in movement and postures. If so, start with a practice in Chapter 4 that meets your current need. As your situation changes, try another practice. If you feel drawn to meditation or yoga philosophy, go in that direction, or at least, set aside some time to explore it. Then you can add that dimension to your practice of postures and breathing.

Where you begin does not really matter. The important thing is *to begin*. Over time, you will probably delve into all the different aspects of yoga. You'll do it step by step, in your own order and in your own way. Studying yoga is a lifelong learning process that continues to expand and deepen as your involvement grows.

You are very fortunate. You are beginning a transformative journey that will enrich your life, expand your self-understanding, touch your soul, and deepen your appreciation and gratitude for every day.

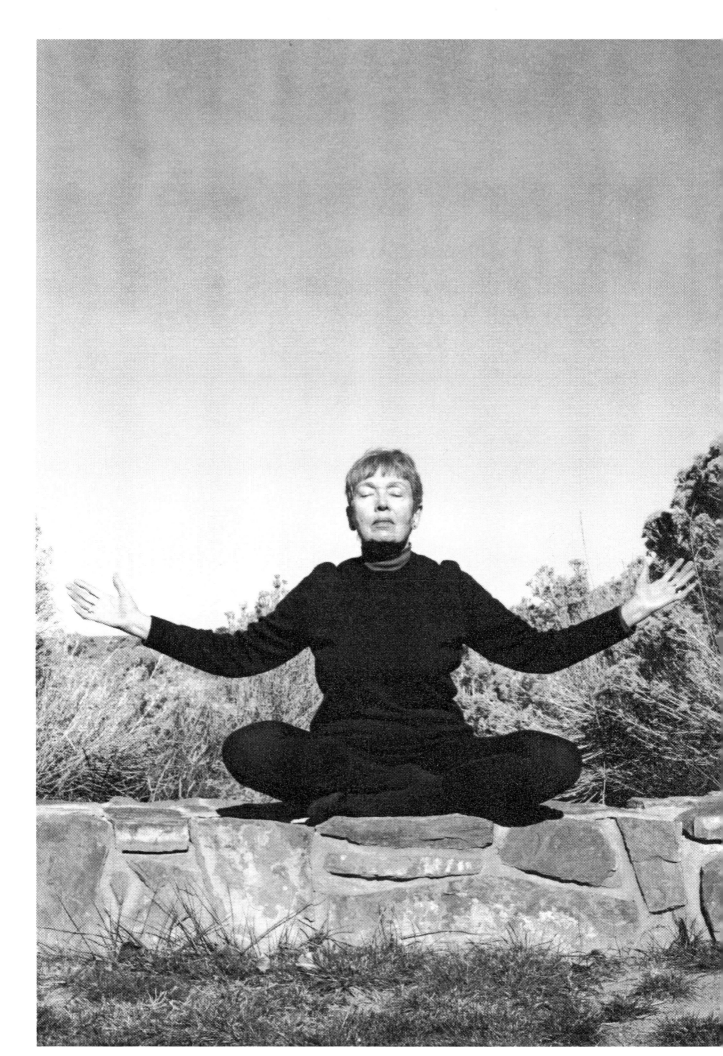

2

Creating a Home Practice

I like to begin my yoga classes with a short, guided meditation as a way to help my students transition from their busy lives to the stillness of class. In one of my favorite meditations I ask students, who are seated with their eyes closed, to imagine that they are a pebble thrown into a river. The pebble sinks through the water effortlessly, letting go of everything, until it reaches the point of perfect rest at the bottom of the soft, sandy riverbed.

I tell them that when they feel that they are no longer pushed or pulled by anything, they will have reached that moment of finding their own perfect rest.

This is your own time, I tell them. This spot where you sit is your own spot. It is on this very site and in this very moment that you can find peace. You don't need to travel to sit beneath a special tree in a distant land. You can find it right here.

And you can create it in your own home.

It doesn't matter whether you live in the heartland of the country, in a bustling city in the northeast, along the west coast, or in the high desert, as I do. It doesn't make a difference whether you own a three-bedroom sprawling house or rent a three-room apartment. Nor does it matter whether you live alone or with a husband, partner or housemate.

What does matter is that you set an intention to develop a yoga practice at home, that you follow through on the guidelines in this chapter, and that you create a support system to help you sustain your practice. The only props you need to get started are a mat so you don't slip and a pillow or blanket to sit on.

As the familiar proverb goes, home is where the heart is. And there is a special place within your own walls that can become the heart and home of your practice. You can create an oasis for yourself without stepping out your front door.

"When I first was introduced to the practice of yoga, I understood it as physical exercise that enhanced balance and strength and fostered relaxation. Within the past six years, however, I have increasingly been led to understand the spiritual element in my practice. Teachers have helped me to integrate breath into each movement of my practice—breath, I have come to understand, provides healing from the divine.

"In my daily practice, I begin with a reading that often provides my intention for that practice. Often ideas presented in class will support an intention. In a recent class, we were asked to focus upon the relationship between a strong foundation in the warrior pose and the grace of the movement of the upper body. I concentrated upon that balance throughout my practice. In the sitting meditation that followed, I was able to focus on the quest for balance within my own spirit."

—Peggy Garrett, 71 (shown on page 22)

The Value of a Home Practice

After you've been going to class for awhile, you may begin to feel that there's something more to yoga than just attending class once or twice a week. You leave class feeling calm and centered. You've noticed you're more flexible and limber too. Even your balance is improving. You can't help wondering: If I practiced more, could I feel like this every day?

Your teacher may have made references to concepts from classical yoga texts, such as the *Yoga Sutra*. Or you may hear others talking about how yoga has helped them cope with stress or how they are getting to know themselves better through yoga. You're realizing more and more that yoga isn't just about doing the postures right. You may have recognized, too, that there's a spiritual element involved for people who are serious about their practice. Any of these occurrences may have piqued your curiosity and motivated you to explore a practice of your own.

Practicing at home is a way to deepen your practice and to make it your own. When you attend class, the teacher is in charge and decides which poses you'll do on that particular day. If you're fortunate to live close to a teacher who gives private instruction, he or she can guide your personal practice. If that's not possible, then you are your own architect. You decide where you're going to practice, at what time of the day, and for how long. You choose which practice you want to do on that particular day. One day you may need more energy; another day, you may feel stressed out and want a more calming practice. Or, you may need a practice to help you sleep at night. Once you become familiar with the sequences, you can experiment with them.

The biggest reason to practice at home on a regular basis is that the benefits that I discussed in Chapter 1 will last longer and you'll feel them on a more fundamental level. As you continue to develop your own practice and deepen it, yoga will become more important to you and more integrated into your life. Yoga will no longer be something that's separate from the rest of your life. Yoga will be about how you live your life.

Making Yoga a Priority

Your attitude toward your practice is a big factor in whether your yoga practice becomes a reality or is just something that you'd like to do someday. You must want to make yoga a bigger part of your life. You may have heard that yoga is good for you and you "should" practice more, but that will not motivate you to do so. Or, if you see yoga as another item on your "to do" list, it will be done mechanically, as another chore to be crossed off the list. Yoga should be something that you look forward to, like meeting with an old friend.

You must feel within your heart that this is something that you truly want to do. The fact that you are reading this book is an important sign that you are serious about establishing a practice at home.

Setting an intention is the first step toward making yoga a priority. Think about how often you want to practice and then, realistically look at how often you think you *will* practice. Do the same with the length of your practice. You might begin with the intention to practice 20 minutes three times a week for the first two weeks and then evaluate whether the length and frequency of the practice works for you.

Write down your intention. Somehow when you write it, rather than just think about it, you give your intention more care and attention. Making a written commitment makes it more real and there's a greater chance that you'll follow through on it. You might even consider keeping a journal of your progress in relation to your yoga practice.

All of these things help you get started and keep you on track. Keep in mind, though, that it takes time to establish a new habit. There will be days you don't feel like practicing and days when you can't get enough. Don't wait until you're "in the mood" to practice. As a familiar commercial says, Just Do It. And you will reap the rewards.

Setting Up Your Home Practice

You can practice yoga anywhere: on the beach, on a hiking trail, in a hotel room, or in a chair at your desk. Once you start practicing regularly, you can experiment with different venues and take your practice along when you travel. But for now, when you're trying to launch the habit of a regular practice, it's important to practice at the same place and the same time. Here are the answers to some questions that you may have about setting up your home practice.

Where Should I Practice?

To find a space to practice, take a leisurely walk through your house or apartment and find a room that is quiet. If you live with other people, find a place that is somewhat isolated from the sounds of the house where others won't interrupt you by walking through. If you live alone, look for a secluded area that you can make sacrosanct.

Ana Franklin, 60, a yoga teacher in Manhattan, Kansas, felt she didn't have much choice in her selection of practice space since her bedroom, dining room and studio are one. She set up her practice area in the east corner of the room. She simply bought a wooden plant stand and put a sheet of glass on top. On it she put things that were meaningful to her: a conch, a candle, a blue glass vase of silk poppies, and a lei of different seeds given to her by a close friend. She always places a glass of fresh, clear water on the stand as well.

In my case, I open the bedroom shades and stretch out my yoga mat at the foot of my bed. I position my mat so that I can view my source of inspiration: my garden and the mountains. The early morning light pours in. Family photos and warm earth tones surround me. I don't feel a need to have an external marker for my practice.

But many people prefer to set up a more defined space for their practice. Whether you choose to do this is a very personal decision. Yours may include a photograph, fresh flowers, a candle or meaningful mementos. You may want to talk to others about what they do or simply do what feels comfortable for you.

Whether or not you construct something special to mark your practice space, it's a good idea to cover a television or computer with a cloth to clear the area of potential distractions.

If you don't live alone, you need to consider your husband or partner's whereabouts in the morning. In my case, my husband is an early riser so after he gets up, I have our bedroom to myself. He doesn't come back in so I'm assured of privacy and quiet. I don't leave the bedroom until I've completed my practice, which means I don't interact with him before I practice. I go directly from sleep to practice without getting involved in any social interaction.

Your situation may be different because of the layout of your house or you may prefer to begin your day with a cup of coffee or tea with partner or spouse, and then do your practice. There is no right or wrong here. It's a personal preference.

Lorraine Schechter, 60, an artist, poet and educator in Santa Fe, lives with her two cats. For her practice space, she chose an area of her bedroom. "This is my sacred corner," she says. "It houses my sacred images and my yoga space." The wooden altar itself is special because it was built by a good friend and contains a candle, a small incense holder, and a little gong given to her as a house gift. She wakes up every morning at 4:30 a.m. and spends the first hour of her day doing meditation and yoga. That time alone, she says, "helps me center and connect with the deepest part of myself, so my day is guided by that wisdom and compassion. That's the ideal. When I don't practice, I feel more disconnected and out of touch with that inner guidance."

How Long Should I Practice?

When you first start to practice at home, it's best to begin with a short practice. Start with 15 or 20 minutes a day. You can always expand it as you get involved and crave more time. The important thing initially is to make a time commitment that is realistic for you to adhere to. Even if it's only ten minutes a day, you are setting up a routine and starting a habit. Once that is established, you can always extend it.

What Time of Day Should I Practice?

I would strongly recommend that you practice the first thing in the morning, unless you have a particular reason not to. Wash your face, brush your teeth and throw out your mat and begin. Practice before you drink your first coffee or tea of the day, before you read the newspaper or talk to anyone. Make your practice a part of your morning ritual.

Some people like to practice in the late afternoon, or just before dinner. Practicing then can help you wind down from your day and transition to the evening. This time of day, however, is often hard to hold to. The afternoon activities or work can run late, you may have errands, or you may want to take a nap. All these things can interfere and prevent you from practicing, particularly in the beginning when your motivation may not be as strong as it will be later when your practice is well established.

The morning, on the other hand, is a good time to practice because there are fewer distractions and delays, and you can begin your day feeling centered and balanced. Your practice will serve as a foundation for your day.

How Can I Get Support for My Practice?

When you decide to create a home practice, it's a good idea to inform your husband, partner or housemate beforehand of what this will entail: which days you plan to practice, where you will be practicing, how long it will take, and so on. Then share your expectations with him or her. For example, you might say that you will not accept phone calls and do not welcome interruptions—"Where's the coffee, honey?"—during your practice time, unless it's something that can't wait. When you do this, you show him that you honor this time as sacred. If he feels informed and included in your decision to practice, there's a better chance that he'll respect your wishes. As with any new activity, though, it may take time to assess what's important and what's not. It may require some give-and-take until you reach a plan that works for both of you.

Don't forget to think about your pets' role in your practice. This may sound silly, but many people have found that pets are one of the biggest obstacles to practicing at home. When you get on the floor, dogs and cats think you want to play. They crawl on your chest, lick your face or paw your hair. You can either learn to accommodate their antics or find a way to keep them out of the room while you're practicing.

Besides getting support from those you live with, it's also helpful to find support outside your home. Try to connect with other people who are serious about yoga and practice at home. You can find them if you take a yoga class in the community or just by talking to friends and acquaintances. You'll feel less isolated and you'll have someone nearby to discuss issues or concerns as they develop in relation to your practice.

What If I Don't Feel Like Practicing?

There will inevitably be days when you don't feel like practicing. Maybe you had a late night and want to sleep in. Or you had a fitful sleep and want to rest in bed a few more minutes. If this happens occasionally, that's fine. Honor your feeling and skip your practice. The next day you'll probably feel more like practicing.

If you notice more and more frequently that you don't feel like practicing, then something else may be going on. Here are some questions to consider:

- Are the poses too challenging and you're getting discouraged?
- Are the postures too easy and you're getting bored?

- Does your practice feel flat, like you're just going through the motions?
- Is your mind wandering or are you just rushing through to get done?

If you've answered "yes" to any of these questions, then it's time to reflect on the quality of your practice and make some changes. This may not be something you can do yourself. You may need to find a yoga teacher in the community who can work with you.

As an initial remedy that you can implement on your own, try slowing down: Move more leisurely, breathe deeper, and take extra breaths between repetitions. Pause between inhale and exhale and also between exhale and inhale. Then, reread Chapter 3 on breath awareness and try to bring some of these concepts back into your practice. If this doesn't make a difference, then seek guidance in the community.

Sustaining Your Home Practice

Like anything new, whether it's a marriage or a house, there's a honeymoon period initially when you feel excited and energized. After awhile, you settle into a routine and some of the initial enthusiasm may wear off. Hopefully, this will not happen with your home practice. A more likely scenario is that your interest will grow and you'll want to deepen and lengthen your practice as you start to experience more benefits to practicing regularly.

But even long-time yoga practitioners experience slumps when they lose their enthusiasm or feel as if they're just going through the motions without putting their hearts into it. If you continue practicing, this may happen to you as well.

Here are some ways to keep your practice alive over the long haul:

- Don't stop practicing even if you feel that you're just going through the motions. As long as you are practicing—even if it feels rote and mechanical—you have the opportunity to link to something deeper by just being present. If you stop, you lose that opportunity.
- Do something different to shake things up. Practice at a different time of day. Move your practice to a different part of the house. Add sound to your practice. Include more challenging poses.
- If your practice feels stale, you may be focusing too much on the physical. Try developing more depth by adding breathing exercises, sound or meditation to your *asana* practice.
- Keep a practice journal. Record observations about your practice and your response to it, and write down questions as they arise.
- Find a yoga teacher in your tradition with whom you can work one-on-one. She or he can help you address your own particular issues in a private setting.
- Sign up for yoga classes in your community. Being in class can reinforce your home practice. It can also give you new postures and sequences that can enliven your practice.
- Attend yoga retreats and conferences. It can be very stimulating as well as educational to be in a secluded environment, away from the real world, with others who share your passion for yoga.
- Read about the practice and philosophy. You can begin with the "Resources" section at the back of this book for my suggestions. Then, if these whet your curiosity, check out your local bookstore or library, or subscribe to a yoga magazine.

When you go through a slump, it may be a sign that you need to re-commit yourself to your practice. Just as some people renew their marriage vows when they get older, you may need to reevaluate and renew your intention. A yoga practice is a living thing and it must be responsive to your life, as it changes. If you've had an illness, a move or a loss since you started your home practice, it may be time to modify your intention to fit your lifestyle as it is today. Don't let this discourage you. It is actually a good thing: it shows that you are alive and responsive and that your practice is becoming integrated into your life.

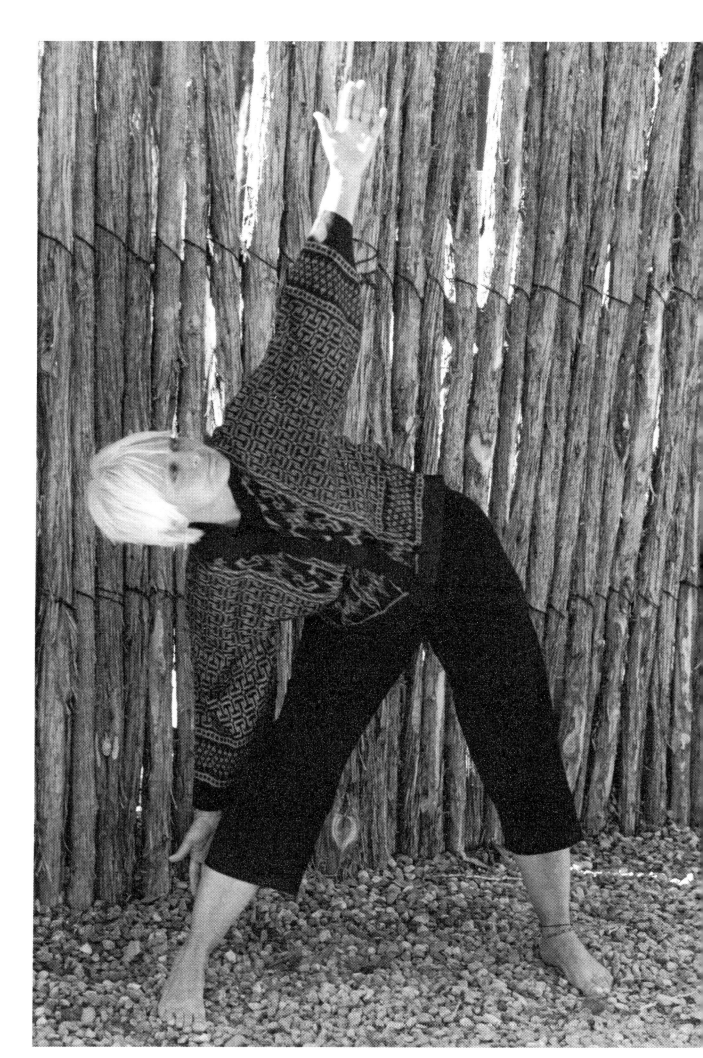

3

Breath Awareness

Breathing is essential to life. It keeps us alive. We don't even have to think about it. We breathe automatically and unconsciously every single day, whether we're awake or asleep.

In yoga practice, we do something different: We bring the breath into our conscious awareness. When we do this, we gain access to information about the state of our minds, our bodies and our energy. Breath is the link and the gateway.

When you're relaxed and calm, your breath is slow and smooth. When you're nervous or agitated, your breath becomes shallow and rapid. In both instances and in many other subtle ways, the breath gives us signals about the condition of our being. It follows, then, that if you can learn to influence your breath, you have an opportunity to begin influencing your mind. Instead of listening to your chattering mind replay old tapes and negative messages again and again, you can learn to direct your thoughts in a more positive direction by focusing on the breath.

When you concentrate on your breath in your yoga practice, there's another advantage as well: It teaches you to stay present. Sometimes we do need to multitask in our daily lives, but generally, it's better to do one thing at a time. Not only does this keep us centered and focused, but we can only enjoy what we're doing when we are genuinely present. If you're listening to a Brahms symphony and writing your to-do list in your head, you can't truly enjoy the music. You won't even hear it. If you're on the phone with a friend and mentally planning your dinner menu, you can't be there for her.

When we breathe consciously and focus only on the breath, we are not reliving the past or planning for the future. We are in the present moment. Once we master this quality in our personal practice, we can begin introducing it into our daily lives. Our lives will be richer for it.

"It has been almost three years since a persistent friend asked me to attend a yoga class with her. Reluctantly, I went and struggled through an hour of difficult asanas. Afterwards, I was surprised to feel a wonderful energy along with a stronger but welcome sense of relaxation and peace that remained with me the entire day.

"I continued to attend classes and began to read about yoga and its many rewards. I now try to practice every day.

"Last December I celebrated my 60th birthday feeling flexible, strong and balanced. A connection of body and mind is created with yoga that extends through all areas of my being. My hope is to practice forever."

—Diane Terhune, 61 (shown on page 34)

Breathing Preparation for Asana

Correct breathing enhances the effects of each posture and allows you to control your breath so that it works with you and for you.

This section will show you how to breathe properly so you can get the most benefit out of your practice. Following are three breathing exercises, each building on the one before it. You can do them sequentially back-to-back, at three different times in one day, or on three different days. It doesn't matter how you space them out, but do follow the order set out below: Begin by observing your breath first, next practice yoga breathing and lastly, try coordinating your breath with your movement.

You'll need ten to 15 minutes for each exercise. Choose a time when you know you won't be interrupted. Turn off the phone. Wear loose-fitting clothes. Stretch your mat on the floor or lie on a carpet and begin.

1. Observing Your Breath

Lie on your back with your knees bent and your feet flat on the floor with your feet about hips' distance apart. Rest your arms at your sides. Close your eyes and breathe naturally.

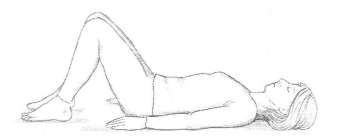

- Notice the state of your mind today. Is your mind racing? Are you feeling relatively calm? Do you feel preoccupied? Simply note how you're feeling without being critical of yourself.
- After a minute or two, begin observing your breath: Is it shallow or deep? Long or short? Smooth or agitated? Loud or soft? Are there any impediments in your breath? Are your inhale and exhale the same length or is one longer?
- Continue observing your breath for several minutes. Allow the breath to become slower, deeper and longer at its own pace. Continue this for several minutes. If your mind is still racing, you can focus yourself by saying, "inhale" as you inhale and "exhale" as you exhale.
- Continue your conscious breathing a little while longer. Before you end this exercise, check in once more with the state of your mind. Do you feel calmer and more relaxed? If not, continue breathing slowly and deeply for several more minutes.
- Then roll over onto your side and take a few breaths there. Use your hands to push yourself up into a seated position. If you're comfortable, remain on the floor. If not, move to a chair. Sit and breathe, gently open your eyes and move on with your day.

2. Conscious Breathing

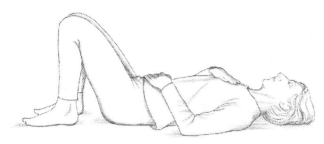

Lie on your back with your knees bent and your feet flat on the floor with your feet about hips' distance apart. Close your eyes. Place one hand on your chest and the other on your abdomen, as shown in the diagram, and begin breathing naturally.

- Breathe through your nose. Yoga breathing is usually done with the mouth closed, unless you have a health reason for not doing so.
- Notice how your body moves under your hands as you breathe in and out. Think about these questions: Where is the breath coming from? When do you feel your abdomen moving? At what point do you notice your chest expanding?
- Take an inhale, then as you exhale, gradually pull in your abdomen below the navel and feel the breath moving upward toward your chest.
- When your exhale is complete, pause a few seconds. Begin your inhale by allowing your chest or rib cage to expand. Let the air move down as you continue to inhale feeling the breath expand your upper and then your lower abdomen.
- Exhale again, contracting your abdominal muscles below the navel and feeling the breath move up toward your chest.
- As you continue to inhale and exhale this way, begin to visualize the circular pattern of your breath. This will reinforce your breathing correctly.
- Continue breathing like this for several minutes.
- Try to pause for 1 - 2 seconds between the inhale and the exhale, and between the exhale and the inhale. This helps slow you down and brings more awareness to your breathing so it doesn't become mechanical.

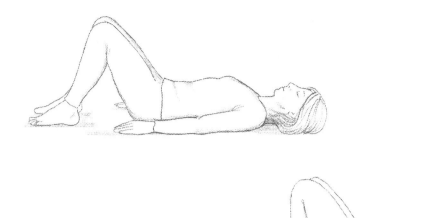

3. Integrating Breath and Movement

Lie on your back with your knees bent and your feet flat on the floor with your feet about hips' distance apart. Close your eyes. Let your arms rest at your sides.

- As you inhale, lift your left arm overhead to the floor behind you. Bend your elbow so that your arm can lie flat on the floor.
- Take a two-second pause with your arm overhead. As you exhale, pull in your abdomen as you lower your arm down to your side.
- Now do the same with the right arm.
- Continue alternating arms, inhaling as you lift your arm and exhaling as you bring it down. Try to make your breath last as long as your movement.
- If you run out of breath before you finish the movement, then try breathing slower or moving your arms a little faster. This coordination may take some practice.
- Lift and lower each arm 6 times. Rest for a few moments and then repeat, lifting and lowering both arms at the same time. Repeat 6 times. Coordinate your breath with your movement.

Does it Matter When I Inhale or Exhale?

When we do yoga, our breathing is not random. It is done in such a way as to enhance the function of the posture. Every time you do an expansive movement, like opening the chest or raising the arms, you inhale. Each time you contract the body or compress the abdomen, as in a forward bend or twist, you exhale. For now, you may need to think about this each time you move. But with time, this pairing of inhale or exhale with movement will become automatic.

How to Breathe in Yoga

Beginning with a very short breath, inhale and exhale through your nose, trying to lengthen each breath slightly. As you do this, you'll notice a soft sound and a sensation at the back of your throat. In Sanskrit, this is called *ujjayi* breathing. It is also called ocean breath because it sounds like the roar of the ocean.

If you're not hearing or feeling this automatically when you lengthen your breath, you can achieve it by opening your mouth and whispering "ah, ah, ah." Then gradually close your mouth while continuing to make the same sound.

Having this sound accompany you as you practice can be very soothing and reassuring. It can also serve as a gauge to the quality of your breath.

Remember to Pause

It may seem like a small thing but adding pauses to your practice can make a huge difference. By taking a two-second pause after each inhale and each exhale, you will bring more awareness to your practice. It will prevent it from becoming mechanical and give you an opportunity to begin noticing in what part of the body you initiate the breath. Pausing also helps you slow you down and stay present.

"As a visual artist, I have relied on my hands to expiate the harsh memories of a difficult childhood. Pounding clay and letting my hands find and form objects, I have been surprised and sometimes shocked by what has come forth from my own hands. For years I thought this, along with therapy, was the most complete and total way of healing the rift in my head and my heart. But then I discovered yoga.

"Yoga, practiced with connection to the breath, has helped me explore myself as a cellular being. What started as attention to musculature and alignment has grown into awareness of the most minute tension and holding, allowing me to search in the nail edges of my toes, in the shin flap on my cheek, in the connection of the bones of my pelvis floor, for any residual cell of memory. Body memory that can then be absorbed and released. Scientists have proven that memory is not only held in the brain, but also functions throughout the body in the synapse between nerve cells.

"The practice of yoga has taken me beyond psychological healing. It has allowed me to actually find and relieve the cells in mind and body that feel damaged. Through yoga, I have been able to make myself whole—cell by cell."

—Leah Stravinsky, 61

Breathing Lessons

As you become more comfortable with the special kind of breathing done in a yoga practice, it will become second nature to you. You'll know when to inhale and when to exhale without even thinking about it. You'll remember automatically to pull in your abdomen when you exhale and to expand your chest with each inhale.

You'll also become more conversant with the meaning of the changes and fluctuations of your breath. For example, if you find yourself running out of breath during a posture, perhaps you're moving too slowly for the amount of breath you have. Pulling in your abdomen on exhale helps control the rate of exhale. If you feel winded after completing a posture, rest before the next repetition. Gradually, try to move more slowly. You may be trying to do too much or moving too fast.

With time and practice, you'll get into your own rhythm. You'll enjoy deep, slow inhales and exhales that last as long as your movement. You'll pause between movements to create a space for added awareness, and you'll begin to bring your ability to be truly present into the rest of your life.

Over time, as you continue to focus on breath awareness, you may feel ready to explore other techniques that can lengthen and deepen your breath. It is best if these are learned under the guidance of a teacher.

4

Everyday Practices

After I had been practicing yoga for about a year, I took a trip to one of the islands in the Caribbean. Transport yourself there with me for a moment.

The sun is shining. It is hot. The water is a deep turquoise. There's a light breeze. After sitting on the beach for a while I decide to go snorkeling. I put on my mask and fins and wade into the water and glide off. The sun is beating down on my back, the water streaming through my hands as I do the breaststroke skimming the surface. I breathe slowly and deliberately through the clear, cool waters. After about twenty minutes, I come out of the water. As I pull off my mask, I say to my husband, "There's nothing there." Then I start laughing. "I mean," I correct myself, "there were no fish."

I had had a beautiful, meditative experience snorkeling and yet I rejected it as nothing, because I hadn't seen any fish. How often we do this. With blinders on, we rush to meet our goal and in the process, we miss the experience entirely. That to me is what yoga is about: Having a goal but also being present in the moment and enjoying that moment; setting an intention but also just being there. The essence is in the balance. This is very difficult to do, but if we can do it in yoga class or in a practice at home, we can begin to bring this awareness and presence to the rest of our lives.

The *asana* practices in this chapter can help you develop this kind of attentiveness while they also focus on fulfilling a particular need. Read the brief explanation of each practice and then decide which one suits you on any particular day.

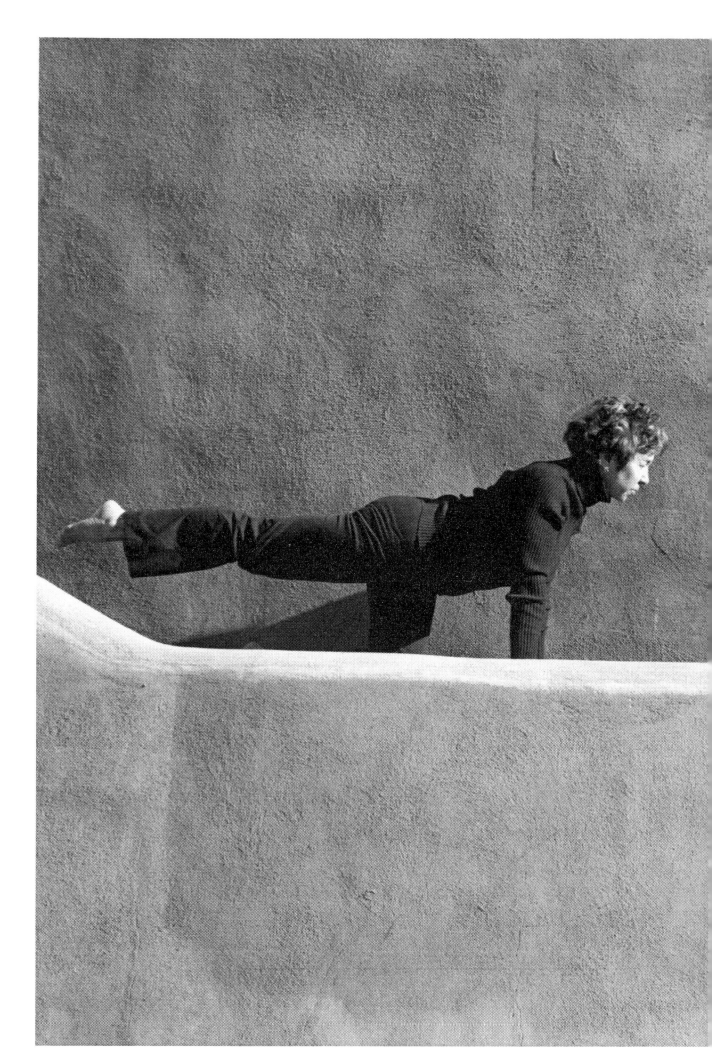

"I didn't discover yoga until I was 48 years old. Like so many people in middle age, I felt stuck in my life and I heard that yoga might be able to help. Without knowing much about what I was getting into, I took the plunge and signed up for an intensive yoga program. My life has not been the same since.

"Hearing people speak of the benefits of yoga and experiencing them directly for myself proved to be two different things entirely. Although a somewhat skeptical person by nature, there was no denying the profound experience I received in body, mind and spirit.

"I have been a practitioner ever since. Celebrating my 60th birthday, I feel so grateful for the strength, flexibility and overall good health I attribute to my practice. But even more importantly, I now perceive life with an overall sense of optimism and wellbeing."

—Laura Feldberg, 60 (shown opposite page)

Before You Begin

Before you start your practice, there are several practical considerations you should be aware of. Keeping these in mind will help your *asana* practice run smoothly.

- Use a mat. It's difficult to do standing poses on a rug or hard wood floor without sliding. A mat will keep you steady and stable. It's also a good idea to take your socks off for standing poses. Bare feet will give you more traction than socks, which can be slippery.
- Do standing poses with your eyes open to aid your balance. Kneeling and seated poses as well as those on your back or belly can be done with your eyes closed.
- Wait one and a half to two hours after eating before you practice.
- Wear comfortable, loose fitting clothing, such as pants with an elastic or drawstring waistband, or sweat clothes or tights. Jeans and belts are too constricting.

Besides these practical considerations, please keep in mind some of the following principles of yoga as you practice:

- Every pose should contain qualities of steadiness and alertness as well as those of ease and comfort. Be conscious of the interplay of these qualities as you practice. For example, in a strong standing posture, your lower body may feel steady and firm while your upper body can feel relaxed and soft.
- Keep your knees and elbows bent and relaxed. Stiff arms and legs breed tension. Relaxing your elbows on arm raises will begin the process of opening your chest while unlocking your knees in standing postures will give your lower back support.
- Rest as needed. It's fine to sit down and take a few breaths between postures if you need to.
- Remember to stay consciously in tune with your breath and to integrate your breath with your movement.
- Pause for 1–2 seconds after each inhale and each exhale. This will bring an awareness to your practice and prevent it from becoming mechanical.

Good Body Mechanics Will Help You Prevent Injuries

- To move from standing to the floor: Place one knee on the floor resting your hands on your other thigh. Then lower the other knee. Shift your upper body to your heels or the floor and then swing your legs around into a seated position.
- To move from lying to sitting: From a lying position, roll over onto your side, placing your palms together under one cheek. Take a few breaths there. Then slide your upper hand out and press that palm into the floor as support to push your body up into a seated position.

- To move from sitting on the floor to standing: Come onto your hands and knees. Then move to your knees with your hands at your sides. Place one foot on the floor and your hands on that thigh, using them as a lever to lift your self to standing.
- If steadiness is a concern, keep a stool or chair nearby for support.

Add Sound to Your Practice for a Deeper Experience.

If you would like to deepen your practice, quiet your mind and become more focused, consider adding sound.

Start with simple sounds, such as "ma" and "so ma," or "ha" and "ha vu." These are basic sounds; they have no meaning. Begin with an easy movement, such as standing arm raises. Inhale as you raise your arms overhead.

Select a pitch that works for your voice. As you exhale and bring your arms down, chant "ha." Repeat this several times. If this is comfortable, you can add a syllable and chant "ha vu." End the sequence by chanting "ha vu ha." You can also do this sequence with the other syllables suggested.

Try to make your sound last as long as it takes you to lower your arms. As you lengthen your chant, you will have to move slower. When you add syllables, you can vary the tone by raising and lowering the pitch one whole step each time.

If you enjoy this, you can make chanting a bigger part of your practice by adding it to any simple standing or kneeling posture.

Ten Everyday Practices

Before you decide which practice to follow, check in with yourself and see how you're feeling today. Do you need energy or calming? Are you restless or sleepy? How much time do you have? Select the practice that you feel will most likely satisfy you on this particular day.

Begin each of the practices in the following way:

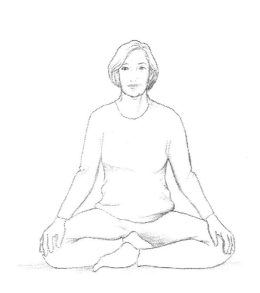 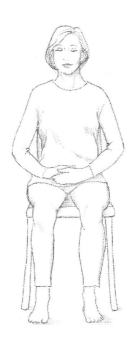

Before you begin to move, sit quietly in a comfortable seated position with your eyes closed. Sit on a chair or on the floor with your legs crossed or out in front of you (not shown). Take a few deep breaths through your nose and exhale with a sigh through your mouth. Try to let go of whatever is going on in your life and just concentrate on your breathing. You can even say to yourself "in" and "out" as you breathe if that helps you focus on your breath. If your mind starts to wander, gently bring it back to your breath. Focus on your breathing for several minutes and then begin one of the following sequences.

A Simple Daily Practice

This practice will serve you well day in and day out, especially at times when you don't have special needs. It's a well-rounded practice that will improve your flexibility, strength, and ability to focus, especially if you do it on a regular basis.

1. Stand with your feet parallel, feet directly below your hips. Release your knees so they aren't locked. Keep your eyes open.

- Inhale—raise your arms overhead.
- Exhale—bring your arms down in front.
- Repeat 4 times.
- Continue with the same movement, coming up onto the balls of your feet or your toes as you inhale and raise your arms.
- Exhale—lower your heels as you bring your arms down.
- Repeat 4 times.

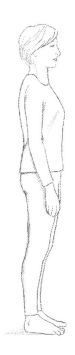
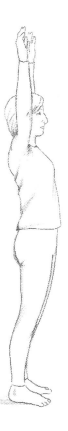

2. Stand with feet parallel directly below your hips with your arms at your sides.

- Inhale—lift the right arm up from your side over your head.
- Exhale—tilt to the left sliding your left hand down your left leg.
- Inhale—come back to center, arm overhead.
- Exhale—lower your right arm.
- Repeat the same movement on the other side, lifting the left arm up and tilting to the right.
- Repeat 4 times on each side.

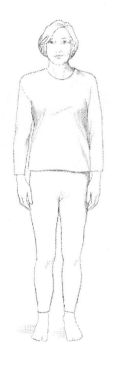

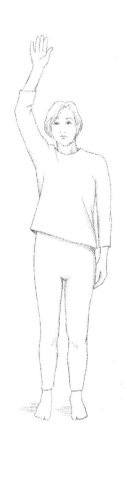

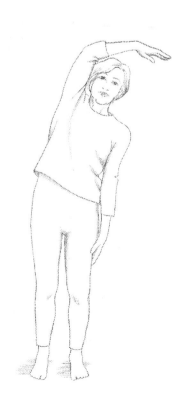

3. Separate your legs so that your stance is wide, arms at your sides.

- Inhale—lift your arms up to shoulder's height.
- Exhale—twist to your left, bringing your left hand to your lower back and your right hand to your left shoulder.
- Inhale—stretch both arms straight.
- Exhale—twist to the right, right hand to your lower back and left hand to your right shoulder.
- Inhale—bring arms back out straight to your shoulder's height.
- Exhale—lower your arms.
- Repeat 4 times on each side.

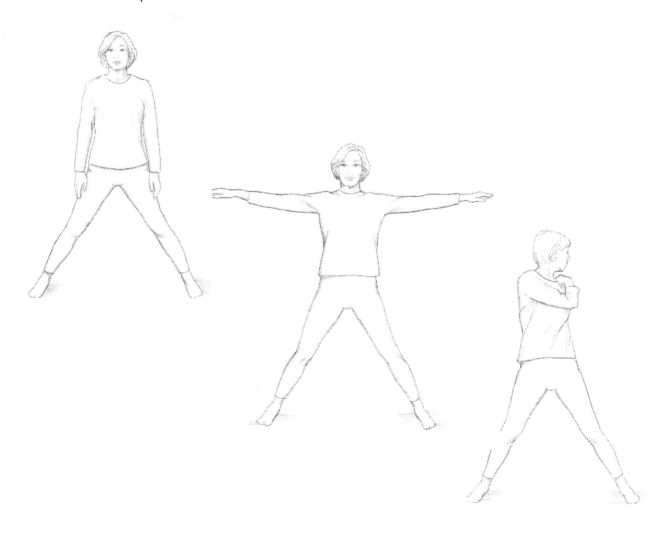

4. Keep your legs spread wide, arms down at your sides.

- Inhale—raise your arms overhead.
- Exhale—fold forward into a deep forward bend, bringing your hands to rest on the floor or on your legs.
- Inhale—raise arms overhead as you come up.
- Repeat 4 times.

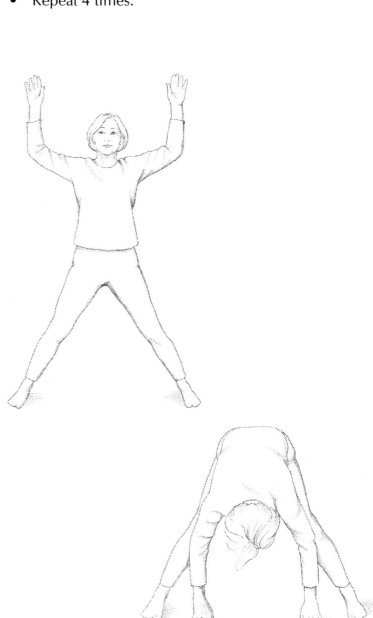

5. Stand with your feet parallel, and then take a big step back with your right foot, placing it at an angle that allows your hips to face forward. To feel more balanced, try slightly widening the distance between your feet.

- Inhale—bend the left knee and lift the arms overhead keeping elbows bent and allowing the back to arch by slightly lifting the chest.
- Exhale—bring the arms down and straighten the left leg.
- Repeat 3 more times on this side.
- Switch legs and repeat the posture on the other side 4 times.

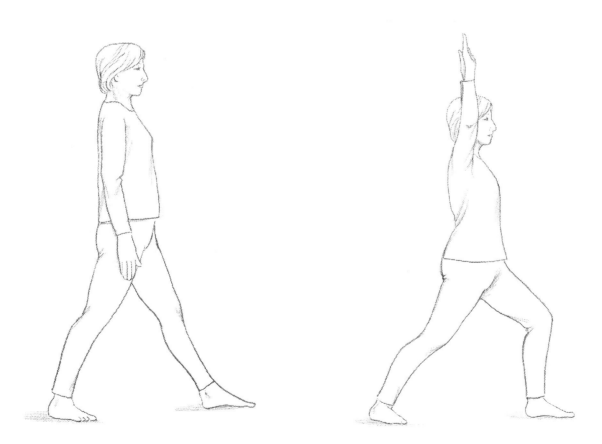

6. Stand with feet parallel, directly below your hips, arms at your sides. Release your knees so they aren't locked.

- Inhale—rest your hands on your thighs.
- Exhale—slide your hands down your legs to just below your knees as you bend forward with a flat back. Your back will be parallel to the floor.
- Inhale—slide your hands up as you come up with a flat back.
- Repeat 4 times.
- Exhale—slide your hands all the way down your legs to your ankles. Begin with a flat back (as above), then release your head, neck and shoulders as you roll down.
- Inhale—slide your hands up your legs as you come all the way.
- Repeat 4 times.

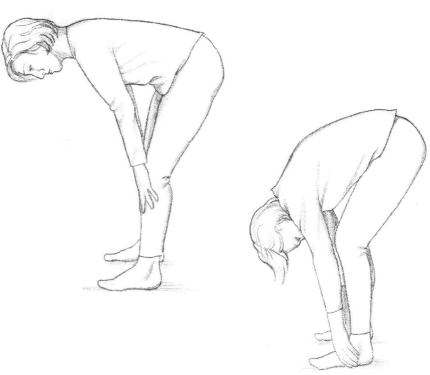

7. Come onto your hands and knees. Place your hands under your shoulders and your knees directly under your hips.

- Inhale—arch your back and look up slightly.
- Exhale—bend your elbows and lower your hips back, dropping your buttocks toward your heels.
- Inhale—lead with your chest coming back onto all fours with your back arched.
- Repeat 6 times.

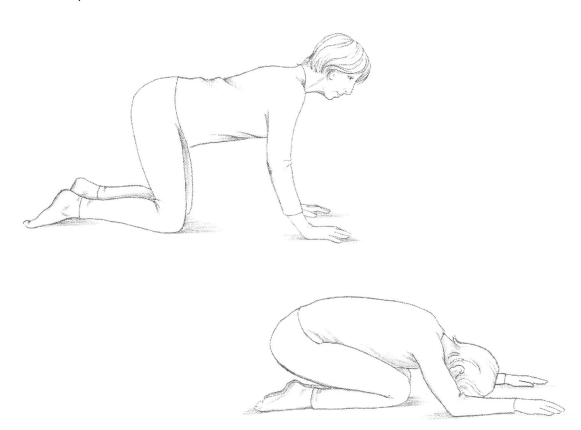

8. Lie on your back with your legs stretched out on the floor or with your knees bent. Rest your arms at your sides.

- Inhale—raise both arms to the floor behind you.
- Exhale—bring your arms down to your sides.
- Do this 6 times.

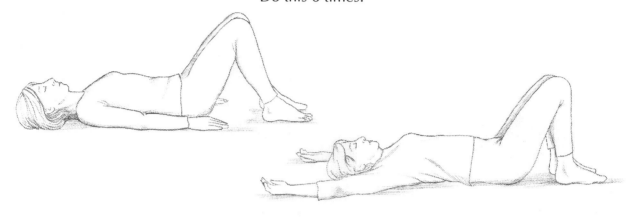

9. Lie on your back with your knees bent, feet hips distance apart flat on the floor. Rest your arms at your sides.

- Exhale—put one hand on each knee and draw them into your chest.
- Inhale—raise both arms to the floor over your head as you straighten your legs up to the ceiling.
  - Exhale—lower your arms and legs, drawing your knees into your chest with a hand on each knee.
  - Repeat 6 times.

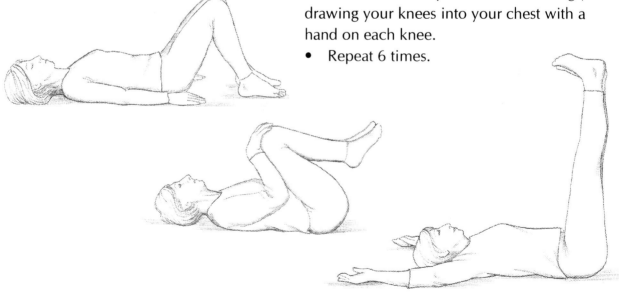

10. Lie on your back with your knees bent, feet hips' distance apart flat on the floor. Rest your arms at your sides.

- Inhale—begin lifting your spine from your buttocks coming up one vertebra at a time. Keep your arms at your sides or raise them overhead as shown.
- Exhale—lower your spine, coming down one vertebra at a time as you lower your arms.
- Repeat 6 times.

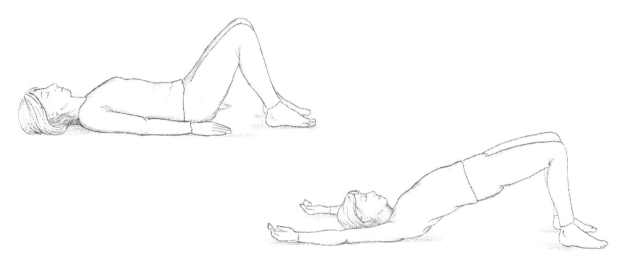

11. Roll over onto your belly and place your forearms on the floor with your elbows close to your body. Put your forehead on the floor.

- Inhale—lift your head and chest off the floor.
- Exhale—lower your chest and place your forehead on the floor.
- Repeat 6 times.

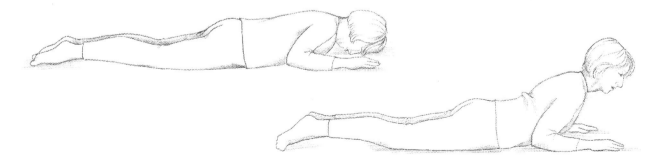

12. Draw your knees into your chest, resting one hand on each knee.

- Inhale—straighten your elbows, allowing your feet to just hang.
- Exhale—bend your elbows and draw your knees to your chest.
- Repeat 6 times.

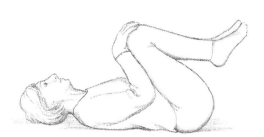 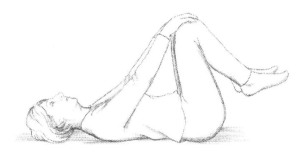

13. Lie down on your back with your legs out straight and your arms at your sides, palms facing up. Close your eyes. Breathe naturally. Observe the quality of your breath. Notice how your breath is moving through your body. See whether your inhale and exhale are the same length, whether you are breathing through your nose or mouth, whether your breath is smooth or rough, shallow or deep. Simply observe these things without making any judgments for several minutes, then let your body melt into the floor. Rest for 5–7 minutes.

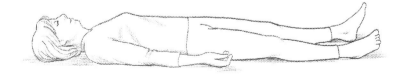

A Restorative Practice

On days when you feel depleted physically and emotionally, you need a restorative practice. Even standing up feels like it takes too much effort. You want to stay close to the floor, move slowly and breathe deeply. This practice will allow you to give yourself the nurturing you need.

1. Lie on your back with your knees bent, feet hips' distance apart flat on the floor. Rest your arms at your sides. Take 8 breaths here.

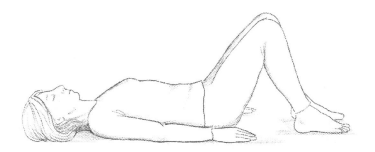

2. Stay in the same position.

- Inhale—lift your left arm overhead to the floor behind you.
- Exhale—lower your arm as you turn your head to the left.
- Inhale—lift your right arm overhead to the floor behind you as your bring your head back to center.
- Exhale—lower your right arm as you turn your head to the right.
- Inhale—lift your left arm as you bring your head back to center.
- Repeat 5 more times on each side.

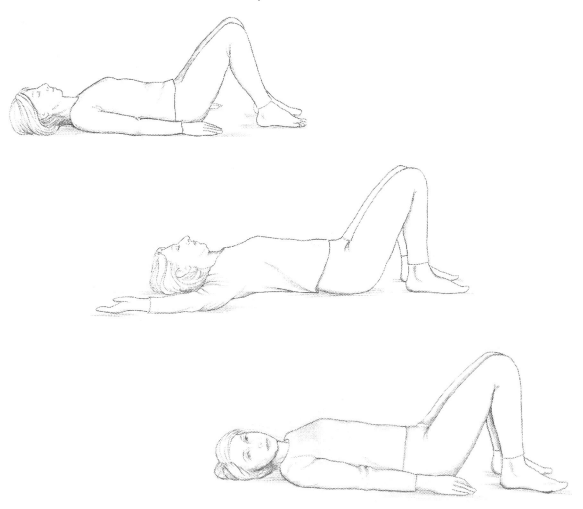

3. Stay in the same position.

- Inhale—lift both arms overhead to the floor behind you. Bend your elbows so your arms lie flat on the floor.
- Exhale—bring both arms down to your side.
- Inhale—repeat 5 more times.

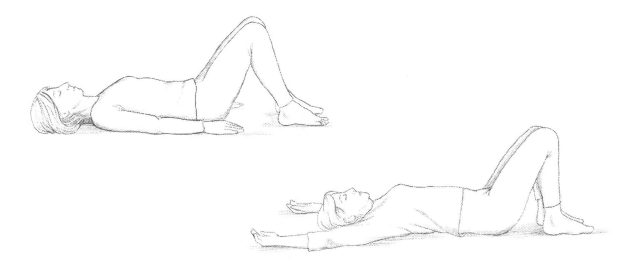

4. Stay in the same position.

- Exhale—put one hand on each knee and draw them into your chest.
- Inhale—raise both arms to the floor over your head as you straighten your legs up to the ceiling.
- Exhale—lower your arms and legs, drawing your knees into your chest with a hand on each knee.
- Repeat 6 times.

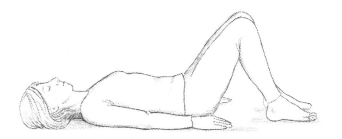

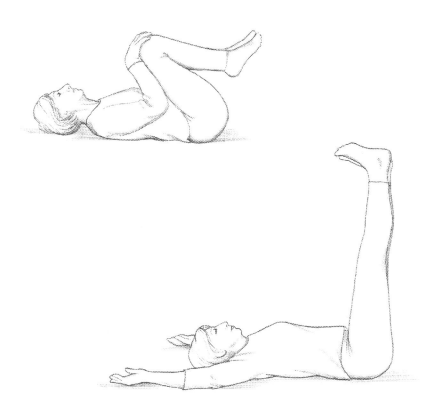

5. Staying on your back, bring your feet in close to your body with your legs touching each other. Stretch your arms out straight, palms down, so they extend at your shoulders.

- Inhale here.
- Exhale—drop your knees to the left as you turn your head to the right. Your knees don't have to go all the way to the floor.
- Inhale—bring your knees and head back to center.
- Exhale—drop your knees to the right as you turn your head to the left.
- Inhale—bring your knees and head back to center.
- Repeat 3 times on each side. Then repeat another 3 times, staying in the twist for one breath on each side.

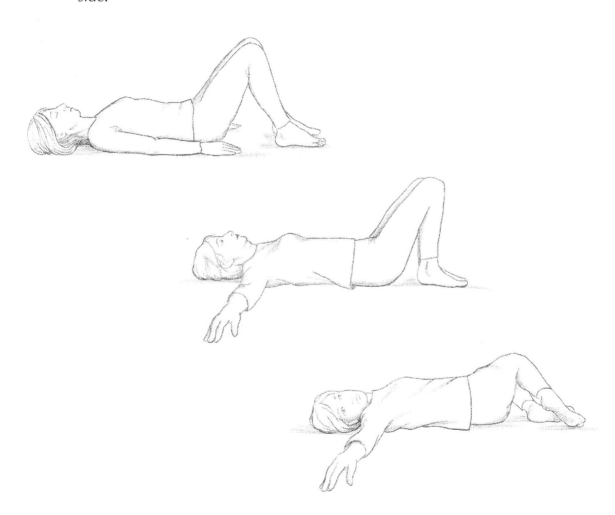

6. Draw your knees into your chest, resting one hand on each knee.

- Inhale—straighten your elbows, allowing your feet to just hang.
- Exhale—bend your elbows and draw your knees to your chest.
- Repeat 6 times.

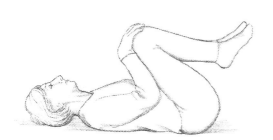 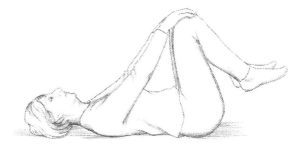

7. Lie on your back with your knees bent, feet hips' distance apart flat on the floor. Rest your arms at your sides.

- Inhale—begin lifting your spine from your buttocks coming up one vertebra at a time. Keep your arms at your sides or raise them over head.
- Exhale—lower your spine, coming down one vertebra at a time, lowering your arms.
- Repeat 3 times dynamically and then repeat 3 times, staying for one breath in the posture.

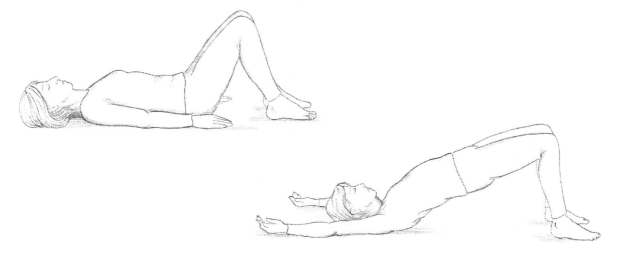

8. Move over to a wall, a bed or a chair. Sit with your body next to the wall and swing your legs up the wall. If you're using a bed or a chair, elevate your legs so your calves rest on the bed or chair. Place your arms at your sides or overhead. Stay and breathe for 5 minutes.

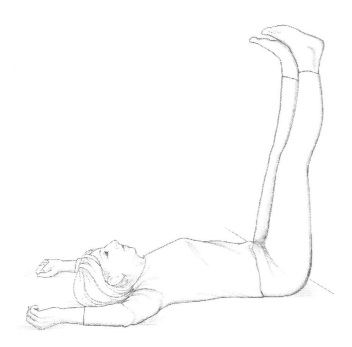

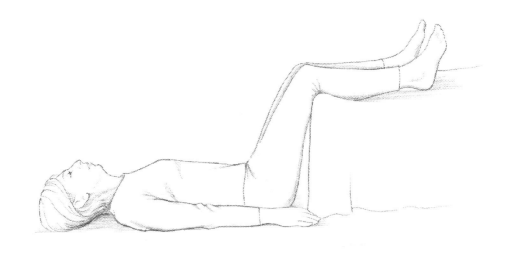

9. Come onto your hands and knees. Place your hands under your shoulders and your knees directly under your hips.

- Inhale—arch your back and look up slightly.
- Exhale—bend your elbows and lower your hips back, dropping your buttocks toward your heels.
- Inhale—lead with your chest coming back onto all fours with your back arched.
- Repeat 6 times.

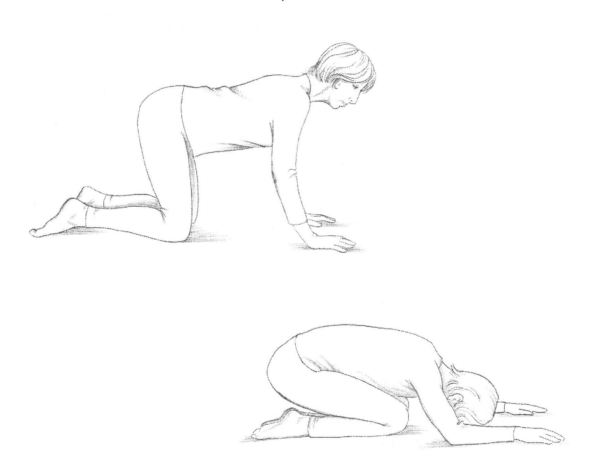

10. Sit in a comfortable position on the floor or on a chair with your hands resting on your knees.

- Inhale—open your right arm.
- Exhale—bring your right hand back to your left shoulder as you turn your head to the left.
- Inhale—open your right arm as you turn your head back to center.
- Exhale—bring your right hand back to your knee.
- Repeat 4 times with each arm.

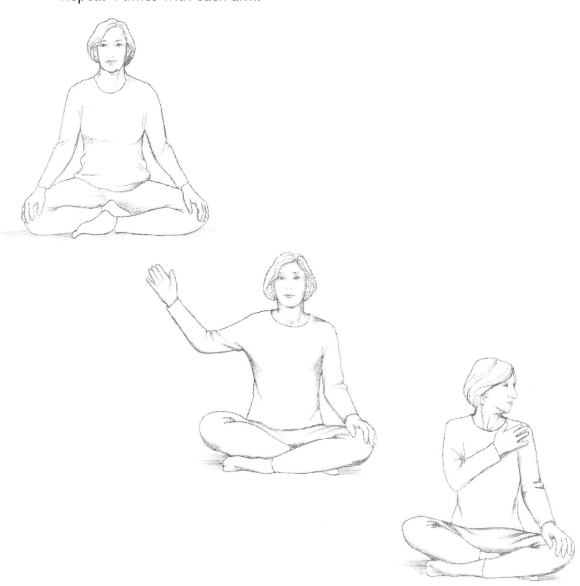

11. Stay in the same position.

- Inhale—open both arms as you lift your head up toward the ceiling.
- Exhale—bring both hands back to your knees as you lower your head.
- Repeat 4 times.

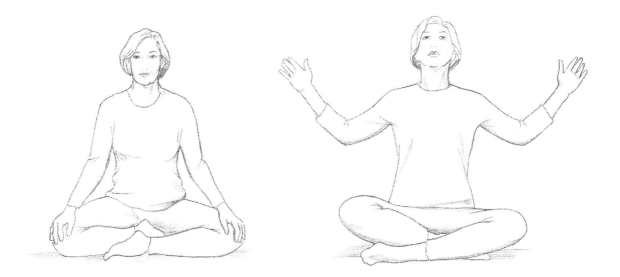

12. Lie on your back with your knees bent, feet flat on the floor with your arms resting at your sides. Do the following breathing pattern:

- Begin with your inhale and exhale both lasting 1 count.
- Do this twice.
- Next, make your inhale and exhale each last 2 counts.
  - With each breath, make your inhale and exhale last one second longer. Repeat each number twice.
  - Extend your inhale and exhale as far as possible.

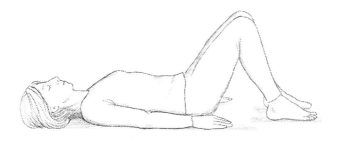

13. Extend your legs out, close your eyes and rest for five minutes.

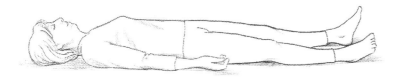

Sequence Options:

1. Do the entire practice: 30 minutes.
2. Follow numbers 1–7 and 12: 15 minutes
3. Follow numbers 7–12: 17 minutes.

A Practice for Energizing

When you're feeling sluggish and low on energy, you need a practice that will invigorate you. You may wake up feeling lethargic or perhaps you need a pick-me-up before dinner so that you can enjoy the evening. This is an active practice that keeps you moving and pushes you to do a bit more. When you finish, you'll feel rejuvenated.

1. Stand with your feet parallel, directly below your hips. Release your knees so they aren't locked. Keep your eyes open.

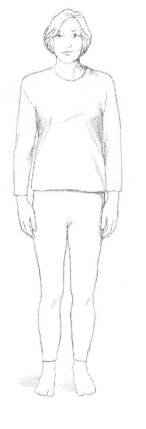
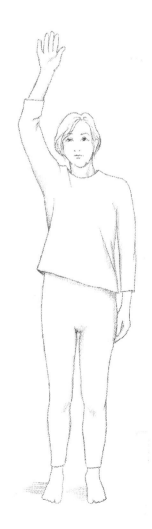

- Inhale—lift your right arm up from the front.
- Exhale—lower your right arm from the front.
- Repeat with the left arm.
- Do arm raises from the front twice with each arm.
- Do arm raises sweeping each arm from the side 2 times.

2. Stand with your feet parallel, directly below your hips. Release your knees so they aren't locked. Keep your eyes open.

- Inhale—raise both arms overhead.
- Exhale—bring your arms down in front.
- Repeat 3 times.
- Continue with the same movement, coming up onto the balls of your feet or your toes as you inhale and raise your arms.
- Exhale—lower your heels as you bring your arms down.
- Repeat 3 times.
- Option: Stay one breath the last 3 repetitions.

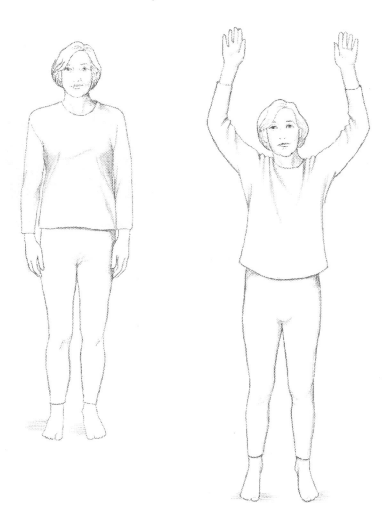

3. Separate your legs so that your stance is wide, arms at your sides.

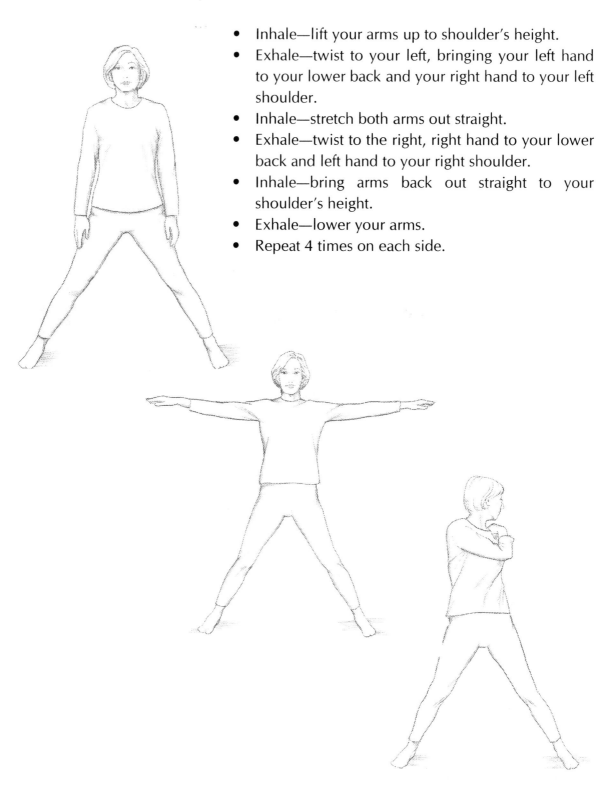

- Inhale—lift your arms up to shoulder's height.
- Exhale—twist to your left, bringing your left hand to your lower back and your right hand to your left shoulder.
- Inhale—stretch both arms out straight.
- Exhale—twist to the right, right hand to your lower back and left hand to your right shoulder.
- Inhale—bring arms back out straight to your shoulder's height.
- Exhale—lower your arms.
- Repeat 4 times on each side.

4. Keep your stance wide, unlock your knees and rest your hand on your thighs.

- Inhale here.
- Exhale—slide your hands down your legs as you move into a wide-legged forward fold.
- Inhale—slide your hands up your legs as you come up to standing.
- Repeat 6 times.

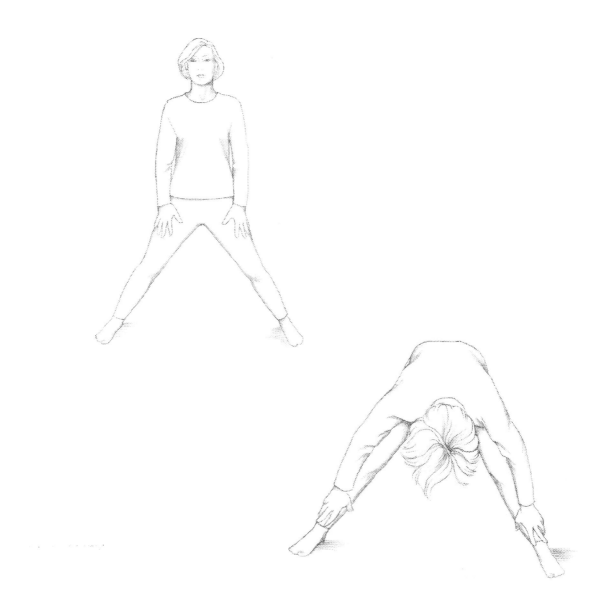

5. Stand with your feet parallel, and then take a big step back with your right foot, placing it at an angle that allows your hips to face forward. To feel more balanced, try slightly widening the distance between your feet.

- Inhale—bend the left knee and lift the arms overhead keeping elbows bent and allowing the back to arch by slightly lifting the chest.
- Exhale—bring the arms down and straighten the left leg.
- Repeat 3 more times dynamically and then repeat 3 more times, staying for one breath.
- Switch legs and repeat the posture on the other side in the same way.

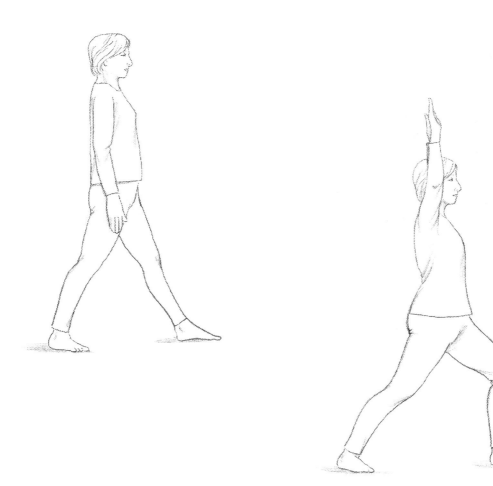

6. Keep your legs spread wide, arms down at your sides.

- Inhale—raise your arms overhead.
- Exhale—fold forward into a deep forward bend, bringing your hands to rest on your legs or the floor.
- Inhale—raise arms overhead as you come up.
- Repeat 4 times.

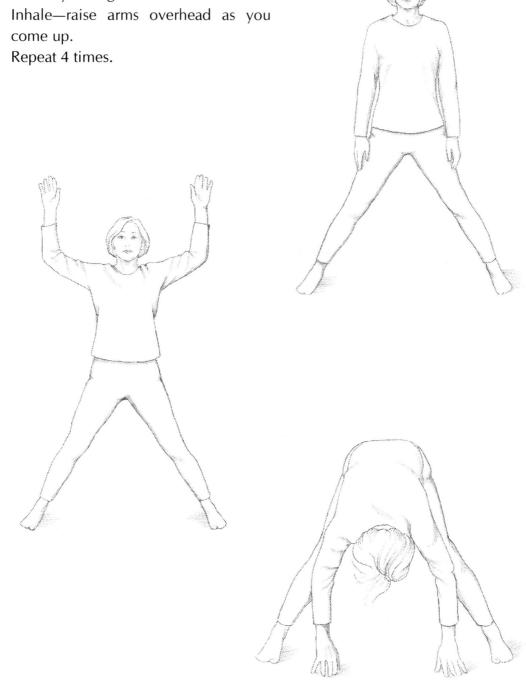

7. Sit in a chair or on the floor and rest 1 minute.

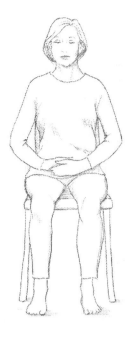

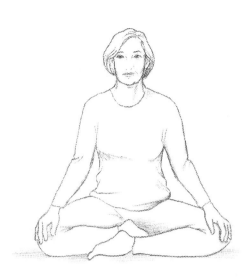

8. Come onto your hands and knees. Place your hands under your shoulders and your knees directly under your hips.

- Inhale—arch your back and look up.
- Exhale—bend your elbows and lower your hips back, dropping your buttocks toward your heels.
- Inhale—lead with your chest coming back onto all fours with your back arched.
- Repeat 6 times and/or continue with the following optional sequence:

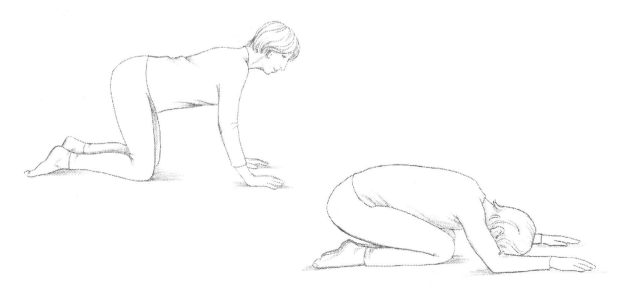

8a. Follow the first three steps above, then proceed:

- Exhale—turn your toes under, lift your buttocks in the air and come onto your hands and feet.
- Inhale—slide your hands forward, drop your body to a prone position with your back arched. Let your toes and hands support your body.
- Exhale—slide your hands back as you lift your buttock in the air and support yourself with your hands and feet.
- Inhale—drop your knees to the floor, arch your back and look up slightly.
- Exhale—bend your elbows and lower your hips back, dropping your buttocks toward your heels.
- Repeat 4 times.

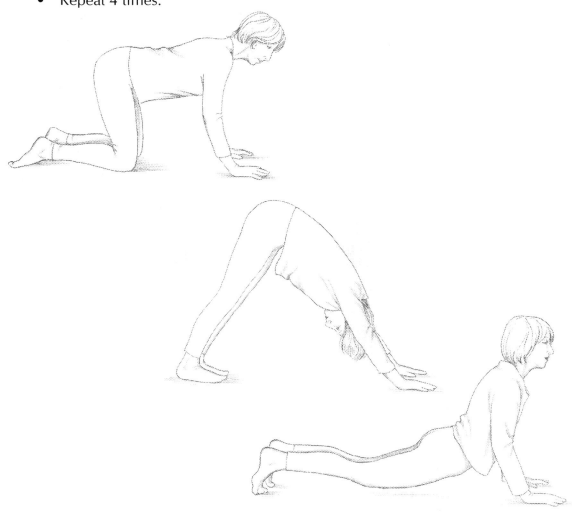

9. Move onto your back. Bend your knees and place your feet hips' distance apart. Rest your arms at your sides.

- Exhale—put one hand on each knee and draw them into your chest.
- Inhale—raise both arms to the floor over your head as you straighten your legs up to the ceiling.
- Exhale—lower your arms and legs, drawing your knees into your chest with a hand on each knee.
- Repeat 4 times dynamically. Repeat 2 more times, staying for 1 breath each time.

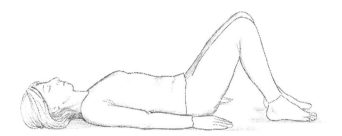

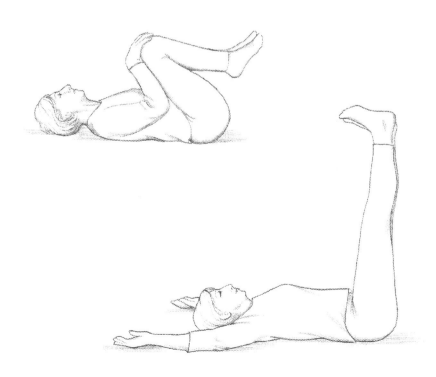

10. Stay in the same position.

- Inhale—begin lifting your spine from your buttocks coming up one vertebra at a time. Keep your arms at your sides or lift them overhead.
- Exhale—lower your spine, coming down one vertebra at a time as you lower your arms.
- Repeat 3 times dynamically and then repeat 3 times, staying for 1 breath each time.

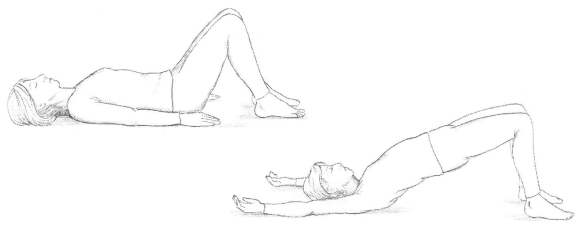

11. Roll over onto your belly and place your forearms on the floor with your elbows close to your body. Put your forehead on the floor.

- Inhale—lift your head and chest off the floor.
- Exhale—lower your chest and place your forehead on the floor.
- Repeat 6 times.

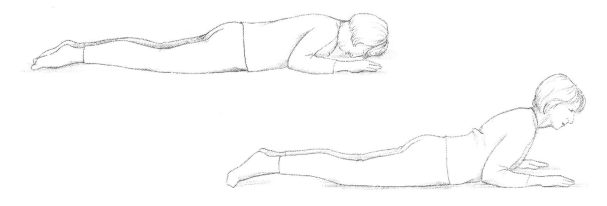

12. Draw your knees into your chest, resting one hand on each knee.

- Inhale—straighten your elbows, allowing your feet to just hang.
- Exhale—bend your elbows and draw your knees to your chest.
- Repeat 6 times.

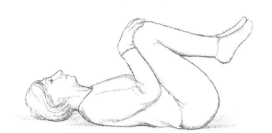 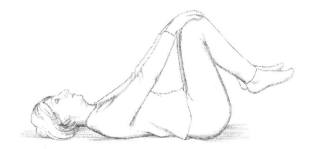

13. Sit in a chair or on the floor and do the following breathing pattern:

- Inhale 6 counts.
- Hold 3 counts.
- Inhale 6 counts
- Pause.
- Repeat this pattern 6 times.

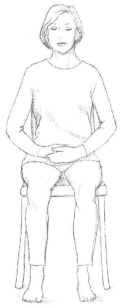 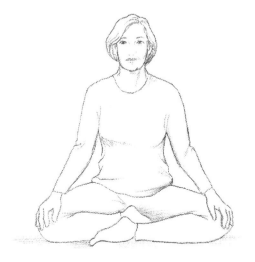

14. Lie on your back with legs stretched out and arms at your sides, palms facing up. Close your eyes and rest for 7–8 minutes.

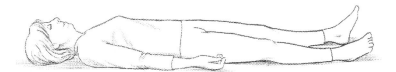

A Meditative Practice

This short, leisurely practice, in which the breath is the main focus and the guiding force behind each movement, is ideal for those times when you're feeling introspective and wish to remain so. You want to move some but not a whole lot. You're more interested in slowing and elongating the breath and using your breath to help you go deeper. This practice is also a good preparation for a sitting meditation.

Choose one or more of the following options to help you slow down and experience a more meditative effect during this practice:

- Start the breath before you begin to move.
- Take a full breath between each movement.
- Make each movement last for a count of 5.
- Pause for 2 seconds between inhale and exhale, and between exhale and inhale.

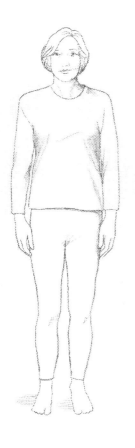

1. Stand with your legs hips' distance apart and arms at your sides. Take 6 deep breaths.

2. Stay standing. Focus your eyes on a spot that doesn't move.

- Inhale—lift your arms overhead as you come onto your toes.
- Exhale—lower your arms as you bring your heels to the floor.
- Repeat 6 times.

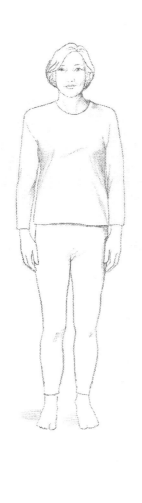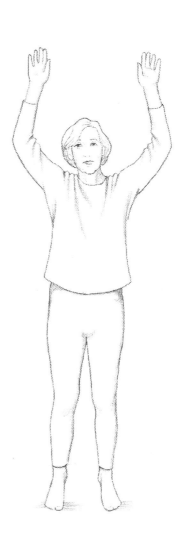

3. Sit in a comfortable position on the floor or on a chair with your hands resting on your knees.

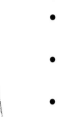

- Inhale—open your right arm.
- Exhale—bring your right hand back to your left shoulder as you turn your head to the left.
- Inhale—open your right arm as you turn your head back to center.
- Exhale—bring your right hand back to your knee.
- Repeat 4 times with each arm.

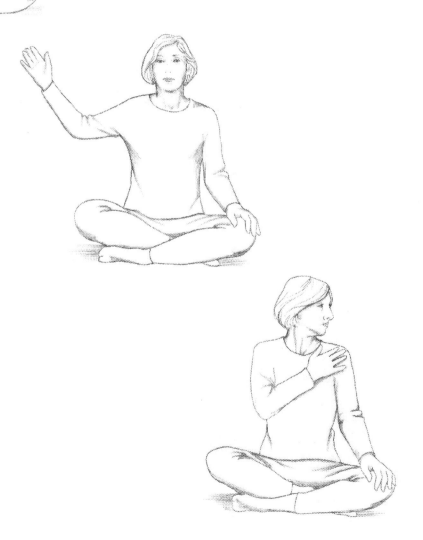

4. Spread your legs wide for this 3-part series.

4a. lateral bend

- Inhale—lift your left arm up from your side over your head.
- Exhale—tilt to the right sliding your right hand down your right leg.
- Inhale—come back to center, arm overhead.
- Exhale—lower your left arm.
- Repeat the same movement on the other side, lifting the right arm up and tilting to the left.

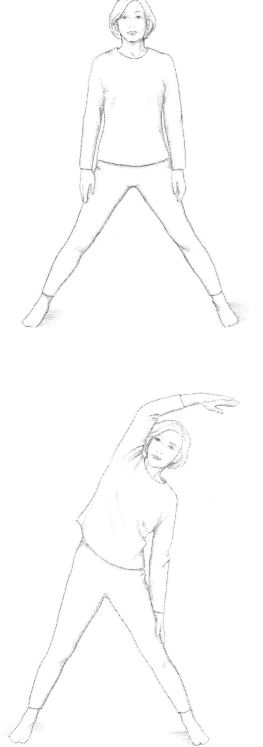

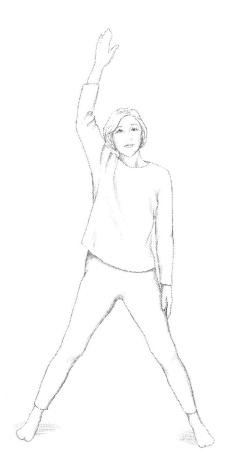

4b. twist

- Inhale—lift your arms up to shoulder's height.
- Exhale—twist to your left, bringing your left hand to your lower back and your right hand to your left shoulder.
- Inhale—stretch both arms out to your sides.
- Exhale—twist to the right, right hand to your lower back and left hand to your right shoulder.
- Inhale—bring arms back out straight to your shoulder's height.
- Exhale—lower your arms.

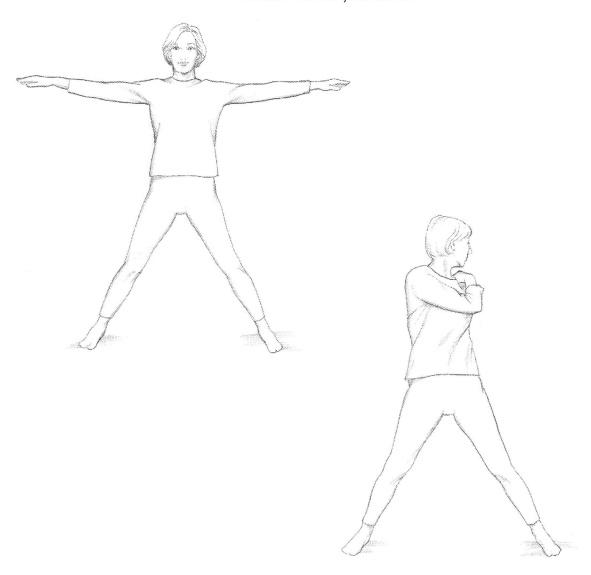

4c. forward bend

- Inhale—raise your arms overhead.
- Exhale—fold forward into a deep forward bend, bringing your hands to rest on your legs or the floor.
- Inhale—raise arms overhead as you come up.
- Repeat the entire sequence 4 times.

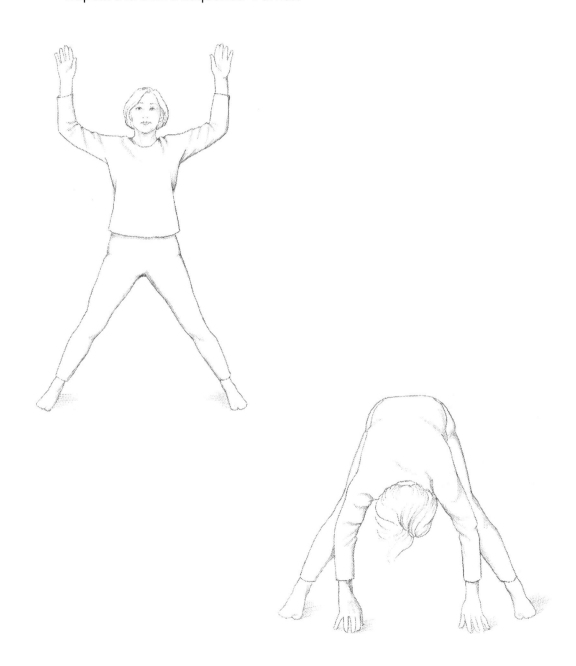

5. Come onto your hands and knees. Place your hands under your shoulders and your knees directly under your hips.

- Inhale—arch your back and look up slightly.
- Exhale—bend your elbows and lower your hips back, dropping your buttocks toward your heels.
- Inhale—lead with your chest coming back onto all fours with your back arched.
- Repeat 6 times.

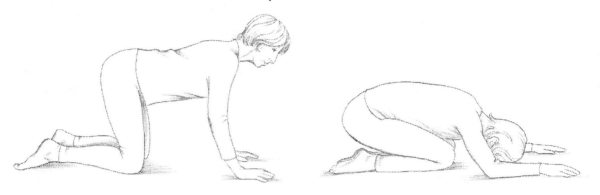

6. Roll over onto your back. Bend your knees and place your feet hips' distance apart. Rest your arms at your sides.

- Inhale—begin lifting your spine from the buttock coming up one vertebra at a time. Keep your arms at your sides, or raise them over your head.
- Exhale—lower your spine, coming down one vertebra at a time, lowering your arms.
- Repeat 6 times.

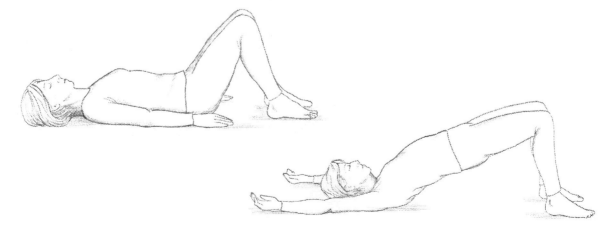

7. Roll over onto your belly and place your forearms on the floor close to your body. Put your forehead on the floor.

- Inhale—lift your head and chest off the floor.
- Exhale—lower your chest and place your forehead on the floor.
- Repeat 6 times.

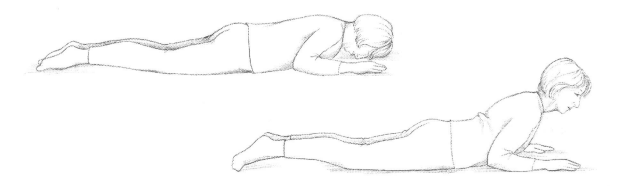

8. Roll over onto your back. Draw your knees into your chest, resting one hand on each knee.

- Inhale—straighten your elbows, allowing your feet to just hang.
- Exhale—bend your elbows and draw your knees to your chest.
- Repeat 6 times.

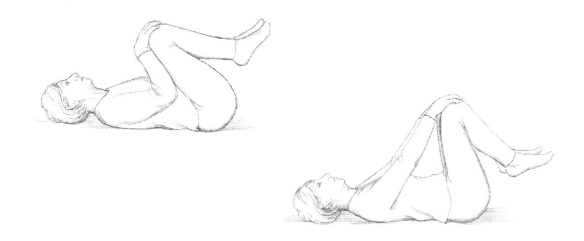

9. Stretch your legs out, close your eyes and rest for 5 minutes.

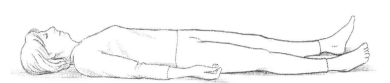

A Practice in Times of Stress

Stress breeds anxiety. When you're stressed, you have difficulty focusing on anything and feel scattered. You need a strong practice to burn up your tension, channel your energy and calm you down. Sometimes when you're stressed, you feel completely depleted. Then use the meditative practice instead. When you finish these practices, you'll return to your life better able to cope with the pressures.

1. Stand with your feet parallel, feet directly below your hips. Release your knees so they aren't locked. Keep your eyes open.

- Inhale—raise both arms overhead.
- Exhale—bring your arms down in front.
- Repeat 4 times.
- Continue with the same movement, coming up onto the balls of your feet or your toes as you inhale and raise your arms.
- Exhale—lower your heels as you bring your arms down.
- Repeat 2 times.
- Option: Stay one breath the last 2 repetitions.

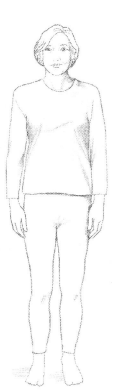
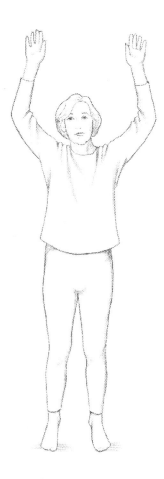

2. Spread your legs wide for this 3-part series.

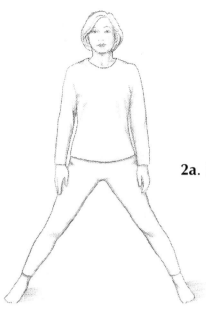

2a. lateral bend

- Inhale—lift your right arm up from your side over your head.
- Exhale—tilt to the left sliding your left hand down your left leg.
- Inhale—come back to center, arm overhead.
- Exhale—lower your right arm.
- Repeat the same movement on the other side, lifting the right arm up and tilting to the left.

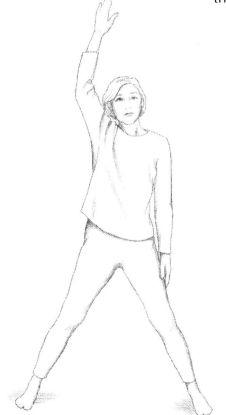

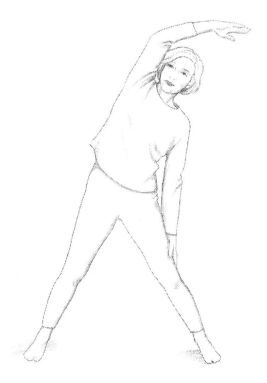

2b. twist

- Inhale—lift your arms up to shoulder's height.
- Exhale—twist to your left, bringing your left hand to your lower back and your right hand to your left shoulder.
- Inhale—stretch both arms out to your sides.
- Exhale—twist to the right, right hand to your lower back and left hand to your right shoulder.
- Inhale—bring arms back out straight to your shoulder's height.
- Exhale—lower your arms.

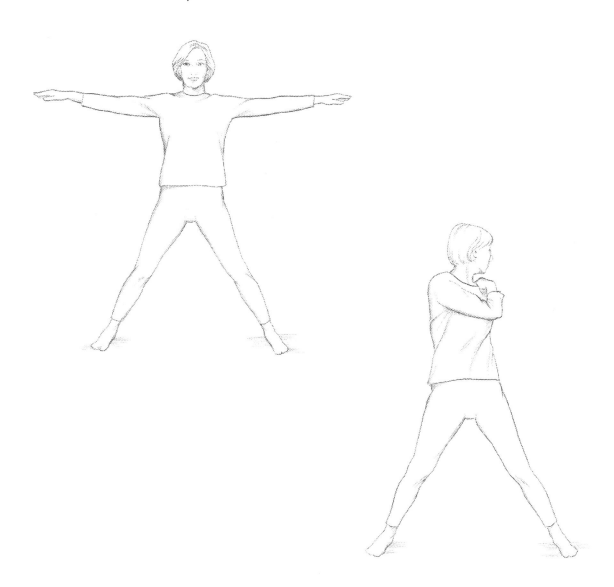

2c. forward bend

- Inhale—raise your arms overhead.
- Exhale—fold forward into a deep forward bend, bringing your hands to rest on your legs.
- Inhale—raise arms overhead as you come up.
- Repeat the entire sequence 2 times dynamically and then 2 times staying in each position for 1 breath.

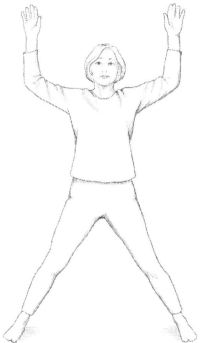

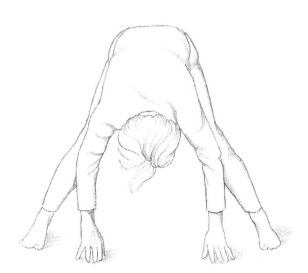

3. Stand with your feet parallel, and then take a big step back with your left foot, placing it at an angle that allows your hips to face forward. To feel more balanced, try slightly widening the distance between your feet.

- Inhale—lift the arms overhead keeping elbows bent and allowing the back to arch by slightly lifting the chest.
- Exhale—bend the right knee and bring the arms down to your right knee or to the floor.
- Inhale—keep your knee bent as you lift your arms overhead.

- Exhale—straighten your knee as you bring your arms down to your sides.
- Repeat 4 times on each side.
- Option: Chant "ha" on each exhale.

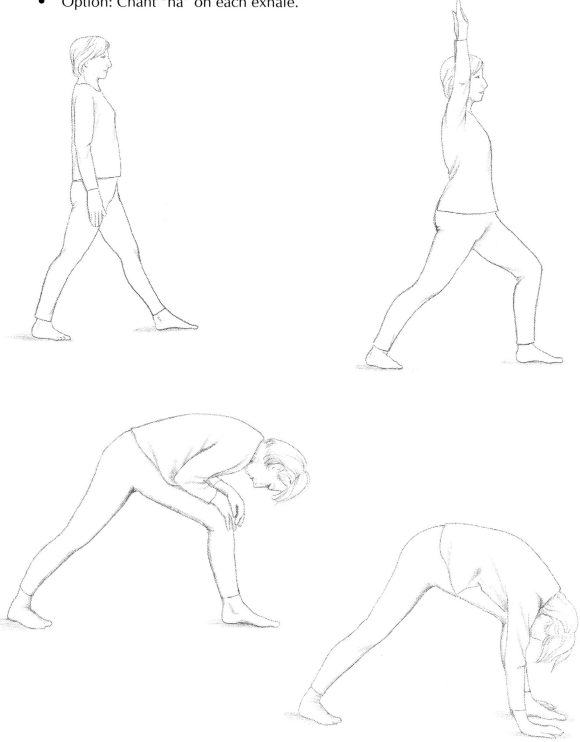

4. Stand with feet parallel, feet below your hips, arms at your sides. Release your knees so they aren't locked.

- Inhale—rest your hands on your thighs.
- Exhale—slide your hands down your legs to your knees as you bend forward with a flat back. Your back will be parallel to the floor.
- Inhale—slide your hands up as you come up with a flat back.
- Repeat 4 times.
- Exhale—slide your hands all the way down your legs. Begin with a flat back (as above) and release your head, neck and shoulders as you roll down.
- Inhale—slide your hands up your legs as you come all up the way.
- Repeat 4 times.

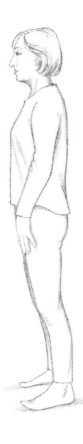

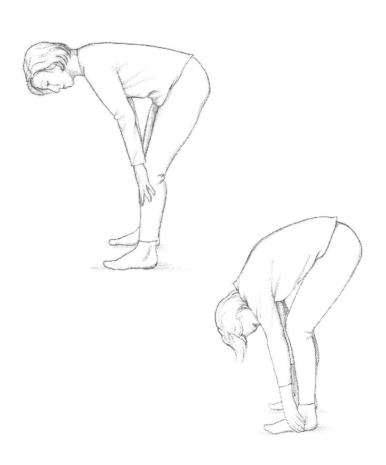

5. Come onto your hands and knees. Place your hands under your shoulders and your knees directly under your hips.

- Inhale—arch your back and look up slightly.
- Exhale—bend your elbows and lower your hips back, dropping your buttocks toward your heels.
- Inhale—lead with your chest coming back onto all fours with your back arched.
- Repeat 6 times.

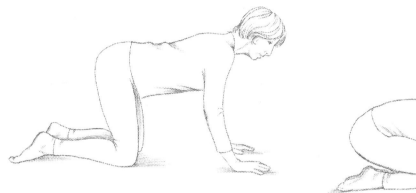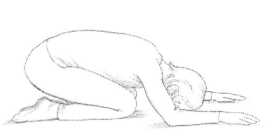

6. Roll over onto your back. Bend your knees and place your feet hips' distance apart. Place your arms at your sides. Rest for 1 minute.

7. Stay on your back in the same position.

- Exhale—put one hand on each knee and draw them into your chest.
- Inhale—raise both arms over your head to the floor as you straighten your legs up to the ceiling.
- Exhale—lower your arms and legs to the floor.

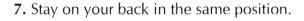

- Inhale—begin lifting your spine from the buttock coming up one vertebra at a time. Keep your arms at your sides, or raise them overhead.
- Exhale—lower your spine, coming down one vertebra at a time, lowering your arms.
- Repeat 3 times dynamically and then repeat 3 times, staying for 1 breath each time.

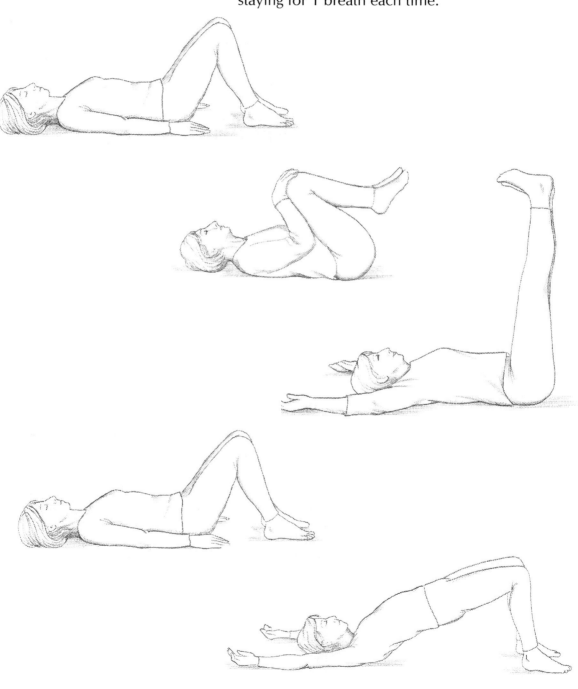

8. Roll over onto your belly and place your forearms on the floor close to your body. Put your forehead on the floor.

- Inhale—lift your head and chest off the floor.
- Exhale—lower your chest and place your forehead on the floor.
- Repeat 3 times dynamically and then repeat 3 times, staying for 1 breath each time.

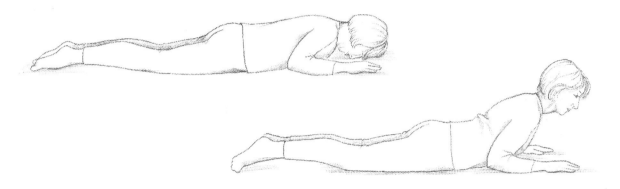

9. Roll over onto your back. Draw your knees into your chest, resting one hand on each knee.

- Inhale—straighten your elbows, allowing your feet to just hang.
- Exhale—bend your elbows and draw your knees to your chest.
- Repeat 6 times.

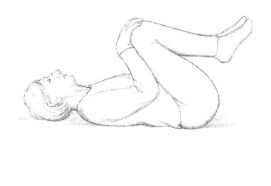

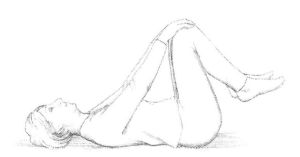

10. Lie on your back. Bend your knees and place your feet hips' distance apart. Place your arms at your sides. Do the following breathing pattern:

- Inhale 2 counts/ exhale 4 counts.
- Inhale 3 counts/ exhale 6 counts.
- Inhale 4 counts/ exhale 8 counts.
- Inhale 5 counts/ exhale 10 counts. (optional)
- Repeat this pattern 4 times. Then sustain the longest count for 4 breaths.

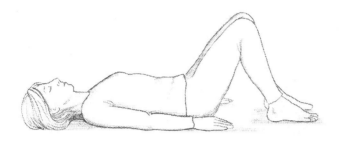

11. Stay on your back and stretch your legs out on the floor. Rest for 5–7 minutes.

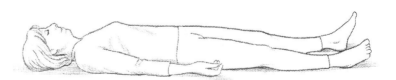

A Practice in a Chair

When you've spent a long time at your desk, it's a good idea to take a break and move a bit. You don't even have to get up from your chair. Just push your chair away from your desk and do this short practice. It will give you relief from the tedium of sitting in one position for a long time.

You can also use this practice on those days when you have difficulty getting to the floor or are not comfortable standing for any length of time.

All of these postures begin the same way: Sit in a chair with your feet flat on the floor and your back erect. Do not lean on the back of the chair. Rest your hands on your thighs.

1. Take 6 deep breaths, making each one a bit deeper than the last.

2. In the same position:

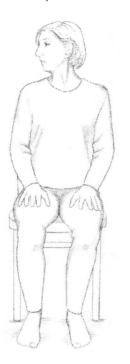

- Inhale—lift the right arm overhead.
- Exhale—lower your right arm as you turn your head to the right.
- Inhale—lift the left arm overhead as you bring your head back to center.
- Inhale—lower the left arm as you turn your head to the left.
- Repeat 6 times with each arm.

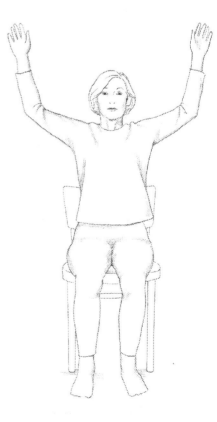

3. In the same position:

- Inhale—lift both arms overhead.
- Exhale—bring both arms down.
- Repeat 6 times.

4. In the same position:

- Inhale—stay here.
- Exhale—drop your chin toward your chest.
- Inhale—rotate your head a quarter of the way around, beginning a small circle.
- Exhale—rotate your head to the halfway point.
- Inhale—rotate your head the next quarter of the way.
- Exhale—complete the circle.
- Make 3 circles, each one a little bit larger than the one before it.
- Repeat in the reverse direction.

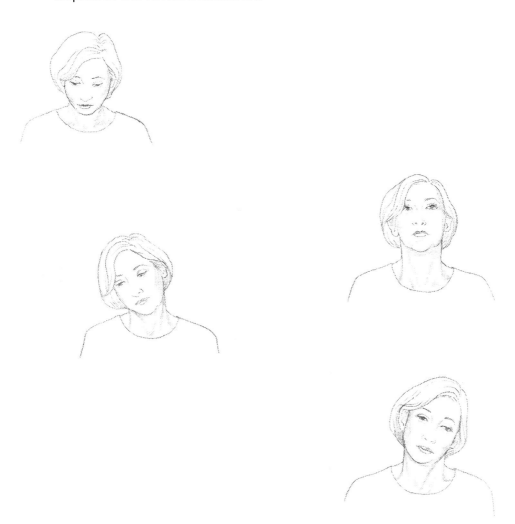

5. In the same position.

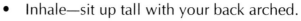

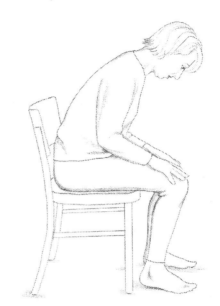

- Inhale—sit up tall with your back arched.
- Exhale—slide your hands down your thighs to your knees as you move your back forward.
- Inhale—slide your hands up your thighs as you lead with your chest and come into an erect position.
- Repeat 6 times.

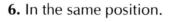

6. In the same position.

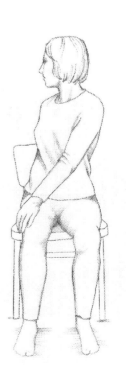

- Inhale—place your left hand on your right thigh and your right hand on the seat of the chair behind you.
- Exhale—twist your upper body to the right looking over your right shoulder.
- Stay and breathe for 6 breaths.
- Repeat on the other side.

7. Stay seated with your hands resting on your thighs.

- Inhale—sit tall with your back arched.
- Exhale—slide your hands down your legs as far as they will go as you allow your back to come forward. Release your head and neck at the bottom.
- Inhale—slide your hands up your legs as you come up with a straight back.
- Repeat 6 times.

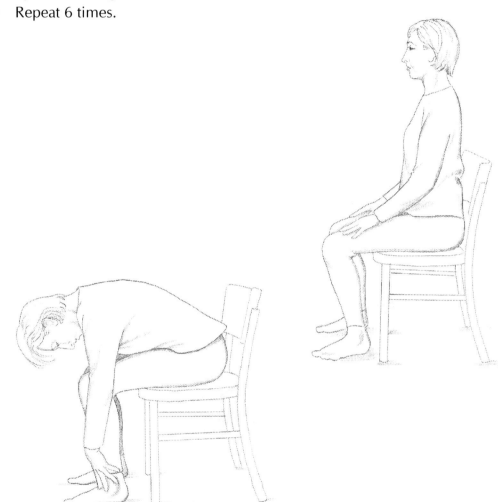

8. Rest your hands on your thighs.

- Inhale—open your right arm.
- Exhale—bring your right hand to your left shoulder as you turn your head to the left.
- Inhale—open your right arm as you turn your head back to center.
- Exhale—lower your right arm to your right thigh.
- Repeat 6 times with each arm.

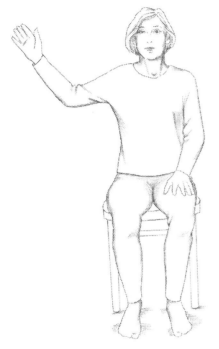

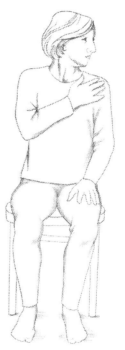

9. Rest both hands on your thighs, close your eyes and take 6 deep breaths.

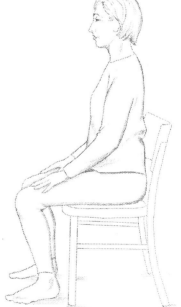

Practicing to a Chair

There may be times following injury or surgery when you want a practice that is more active than one done in a chair, but for physical reasons, you need to be more cautious or you need help balancing. The following practice, based on modifying and adapting standing postures, is designed for that purpose.

1. Stand next to a chair with a high back. Rest your right hand on the back of the chair.

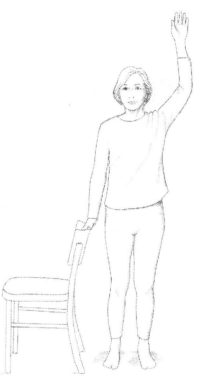

- Inhale—lift your left arm overhead from the front.
- Exhale—lower your left arm as you turn your head to the right.
- Inhale—lift your left arm as you turn your head back to center.
- Exhale—lower your left arm, as you turn your head to the right again.
- Repeat 6 times with your left arm.
- Turn around and rest your left arm on the back of the chair.
- Repeat head turns 6 times with right arm lifts.

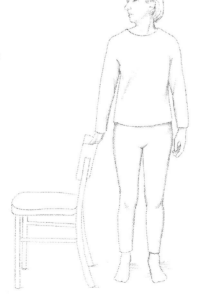

2. Rest one hand on the back of the chair.

- Inhale—come on to your toes.
- Exhale—lower your heels to the floor.
- Repeat 6 times.

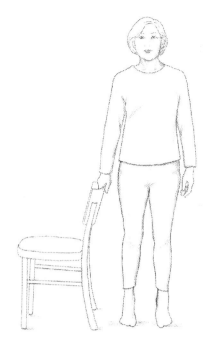

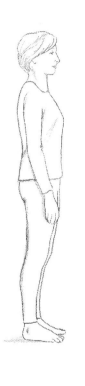

3. Stand facing the chair with your feet about 2 feet away from the chair.

- Inhale—lift your arms overhead.
- Exhale—lower your arms to the back of the chair.
- Inhale—lift your arms overhead as you come up with a flat back.
- Exhale—lower your arms to your sides.
- Repeat 6 times.

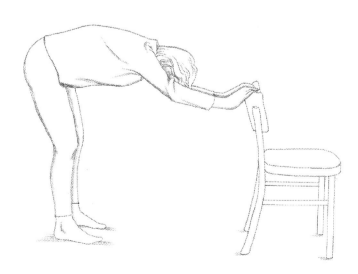

4. Turn the chair around and stand facing the seat of the chair with your feet about 2 feet from the seat.

- Inhale—lift your arms overhead.
- Exhale—lower your arms to the seat of the chair.
- Inhale—lift your arms overhead as you come up with a flat back.
- Exhale—lower your arms to your sides.
- Repeat 6 times.

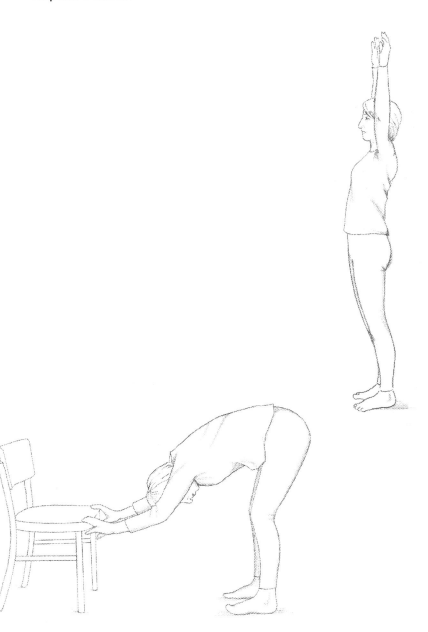
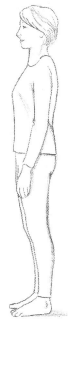

5. Continue standing facing the seat of the chair. Take a big step back with your right foot, placing it at an angle that allows your hips to face forward. To feel more balanced, try slightly widening the distance between your feet.

- Inhale—raise your arms overhead.
- Exhale—bend your left knee as you lower your arms to the seat of the chair.
- Inhale—lift the arms overhead keeping elbows bent and straighten the left leg.
- Exhale—lower your arms to your sides.
- Repeat 3 more times on this side.
- Switch legs and repeat the posture on the other side 4 times.

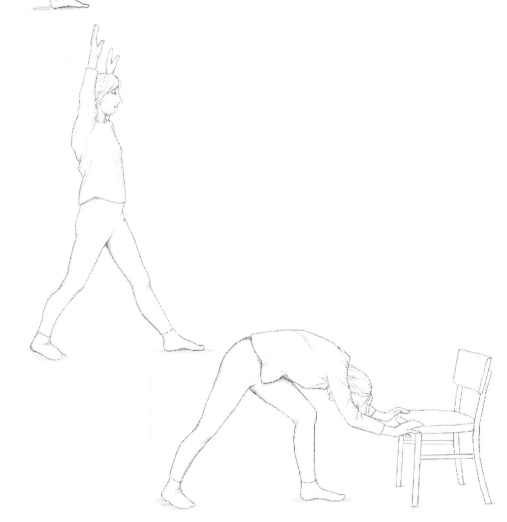

6. Stand next to the back of the chair and rest your right hand on its back.

- Shift your weight to your right leg as you lift your left heel off the floor.
- Focus on a spot on the floor that doesn't move.
- Lift your left foot and put it someplace along your right leg, either above or below your knee.
- Stay and take 6 breaths.
- Turn around and rest your left hand on the back of the chair and repeat the posture standing on your left leg.
- Stay and take 6 breaths.

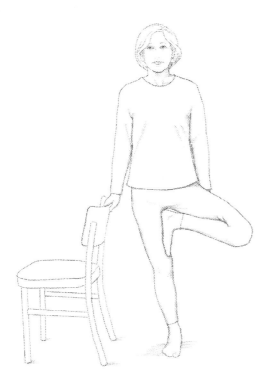

7. Sit in the chair and rest with your eyes closed for 5 minutes.

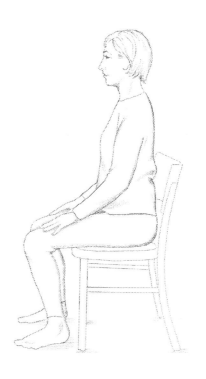

A Practice for Insomnia

Even if you're doing all the right things, such as eating a healthy diet and exercising, there will be days when you can't fall asleep. You may be overtired, experiencing hot flashes, or have a mind that just won't quiet down. These situations call for a special practice. You can utilize the following practice before going to bed to help you relax. You can also use it as an aid to relaxation if you get in bed and can't sleep after 15 or 20 minutes, or if you wake up in the middle of the night with your mind buzzing.

1. Sit on the edge of your bed and take 12 breaths. Observe your breath focusing on pulling your abdomen in on exhale.

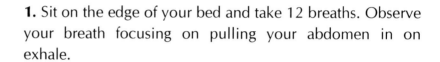

2. Come onto your hands and knees. Place your hands under your shoulders and your knees directly under your hips.

- Inhale—arch your back and look up slightly.
- Exhale—bend your elbows and lower your hips back, dropping your buttocks toward your heels.
- Inhale—lead with your chest coming back onto all fours with your back arched.
- Repeat 6 times.

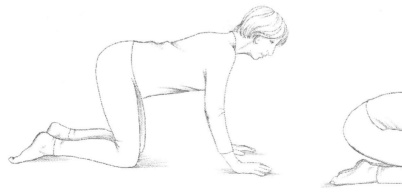

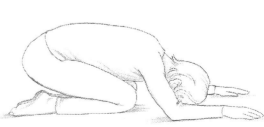

3. Lie on your back with your knees bent and your feet flat on the floor about hips' width apart.

- Inhale—open your arms out on the floor with your elbows bent.
- Exhale—bring your right arm to your left shoulder as you turn your head to the left.
- Inhale—bring your right arm back to the floor.
- Exhale—bring your left arm to your right shoulder as you turn your head to the right.
- Inhale—bring your left arm back to the floor.
- Do this 3 times to each side.
- Repeat 3 more times dropping your knees in the opposite direction of your head turns. Your knees don't have to go all the way to the floor.

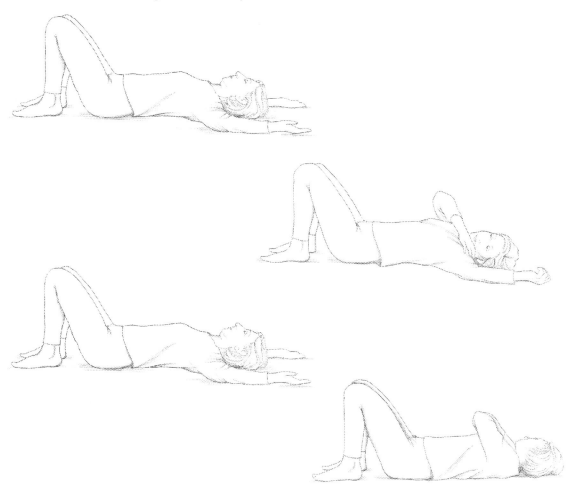

4. Stay on your back with your knees bent and your feet flat on the floor. Rest your arms at your sides.

- Place your left hand on your left knee as you draw it into your chest.
- Inhale—slide your hand up your thigh as your foot gently drops almost to the floor.
- Exhale—slide your hand up your thigh to your knee as you draw you knee into your chest.
- Repeat 6 times on this leg and 6 times on the other leg.

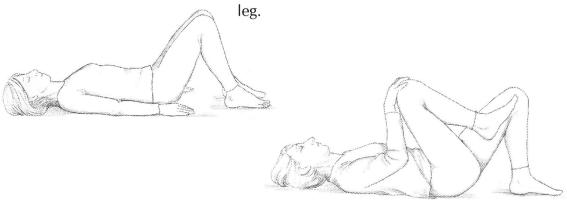

5. Draw your knees into your chest, resting one hand on each knee.

- Inhale—straighten your elbows, allowing your feet to just hang.
- Exhale—bend your elbows and draw your knees to your chest.
- Repeat 4 times.

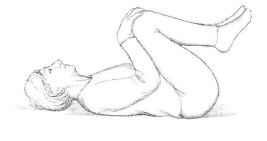
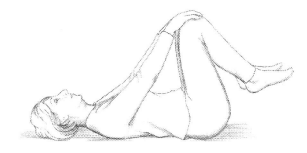

6. Move to your bed and lie down. Start with your knees bent and your feet flat on the bed. Rest your hands on your abdomen and do some deep abdominal breathing for 1–2 minutes. Then,

- Inhale—free
- Exhale—begin your exhale at 2 counts and add one count for each successive breath until you reach 8 counts.
- Keep your exhale at 8 counts for 8 breaths.
- Continue breathing and reduce your exhale back from 8 to 2. Keep your inhale free.
- Repeat 2–3 times or until you fall asleep.

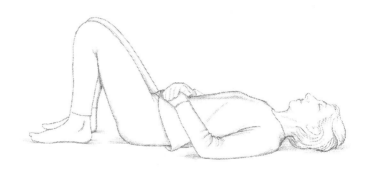

7. Stretch your legs out and go to sleep.

If you experience insomnia in the middle of the night and don't want to get out of bed, do #6 as you lie in bed.

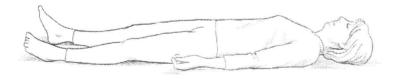

A Ten-Minute Practice

There are many uses for this short practice: You have more than five minutes but don't have enough time for a 25 or 30-minute practice. Perhaps you're traveling or experiencing a very busy period at home. You want to sustain your practice and keep up the momentum but just don't have time for your usual full practice. This short practice will serve that purpose.

1. Lie on your back with your knees bent and take 6 deep breaths.

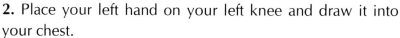

2. Place your left hand on your left knee and draw it into your chest.

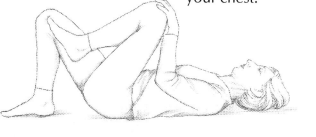

- Inhale—raise the left hand overhead to the floor behind you as you straighten your left leg up to the ceiling.
- Exhale—bring your hand to your knee and your knee to your chest.
- Repeat 6 times.
- Repeat the same movement with the other leg and hand.

3. Draw both knees into your chest with one hand on each knee.

- Inhale—raise both arms overhead to the floor behind you as you straighten your legs up toward the ceiling.
- Exhale—bring your hands to your knees and your knees to your chest.
- Repeat 6 times.

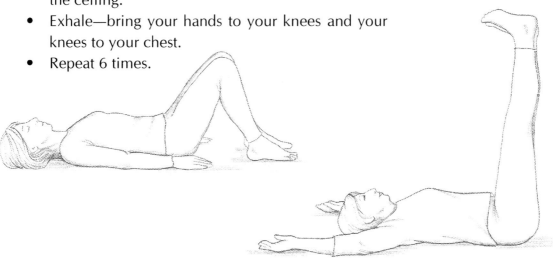

4. Lie on your back with your knees bent, feet hips' distance apart flat on the floor. Rest your arms at your sides.

- Inhale—begin lifting your spine from your buttocks coming up one vertebra at a time. Keep your arms at your sides or raise them overhead.
- Exhale—lower your spine, coming down one vertebra at a time, lowering your arms.
- Repeat 6 times.

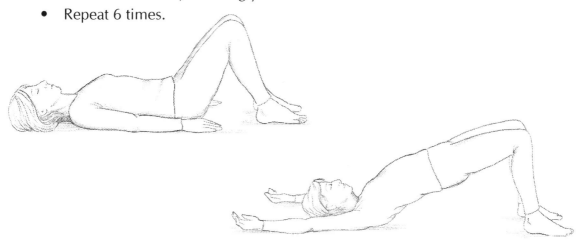

5. Draw your knees into your chest, resting one hand on each knee.

- Inhale—straighten your elbows, allowing your feet to just hang.
- Exhale—bend your elbows and draw your knees to your chest.
- Repeat 6 times.

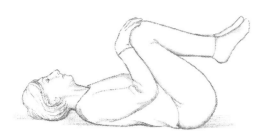 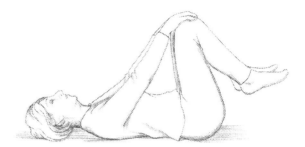

6. Staying on your back, bring your feet in close to your body with your legs touching each other. Stretch your arms out straight, palms down, so they extend at your shoulders.

- Inhale here.
- Exhale—drop your knees to the left as you turn your head to the right. Your knees don't have to go all the way to the floor.
    - Inhale—bring your knees and head back to center.
    - Exhale—drop your knees to the right as you turn your head to the left.
    - Inhale—bring your knees and head back to center.
    - Repeat 6 times on each side.

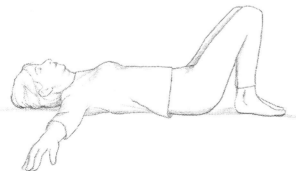

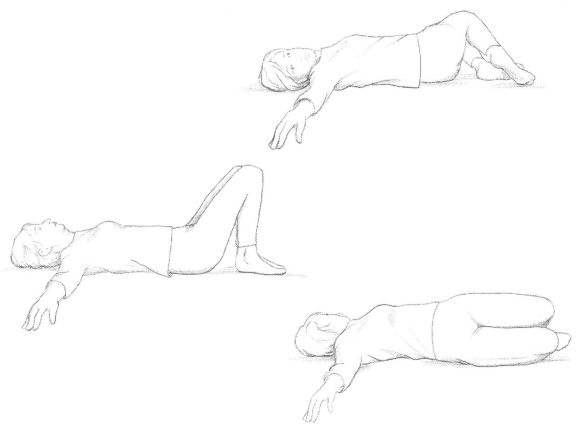

7. Draw your knees into your chest, resting one hand on each knee.

- Inhale—straighten your elbows, allowing your feet to just hang.
- Exhale—bend your elbows and draw your knees to your chest.
- Repeat 4 times.

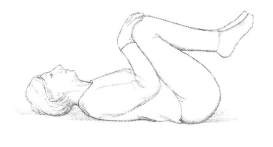

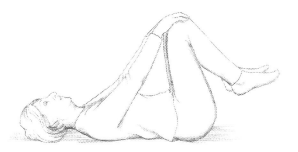

8. Come onto your hands and knees. Place your hands under your shoulders and your knees directly under your hips.

- Inhale—arch your back and look up slightly.
- Exhale—bend your elbows and lower your hips back, dropping your buttocks toward your heels.
- Inhale—lead with your chest coming back onto all fours with your back arched.
- Repeat 6 times.

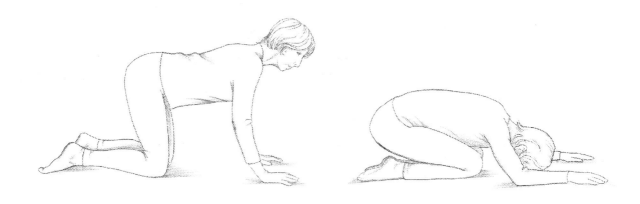

9. Sit on the floor or in a chair and rest with your eyes closed for 1 minute.

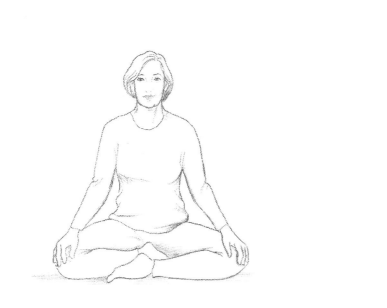
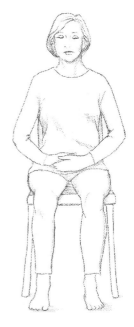

A Five-Minute Practice

Sometimes you have just five minutes to pull yourself together. You need to center yourself before you go out for the evening or focus before giving a presentation or confronting a difficult situation. This mini-practice will do just that.

1. Sit in a chair or in a comfortable position on the floor. Take 12 breaths noticing whether your breath is long or short, smooth or ragged, deep or shallow, and calm or agitated. Work to deepen and elongate your breath.

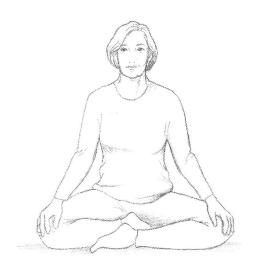

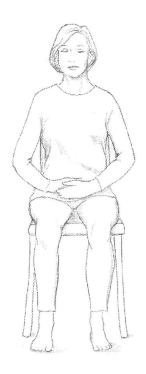

2. Stay seated with your hands resting on your knees.

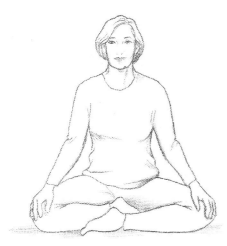

- Inhale—open your right arm.
- Exhale—bring your right hand to your left shoulder as you turn your head to the left.
- Inhale—open your right arm as you turn your head back to center.
- Exhale—bring your right hand back to your knee.
- Alternate arms, repeating 4 times with each arm.

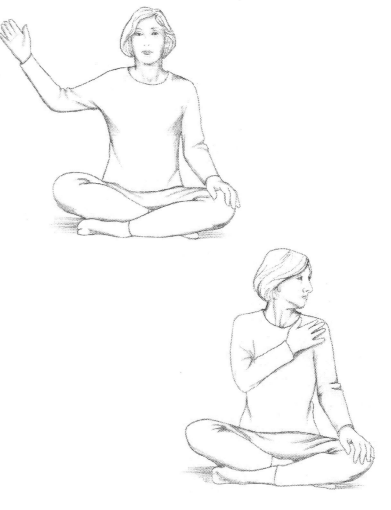

3. Stay in the same position.

- Inhale—open both arms as you lift your head up toward the ceiling.
- Exhale—bring both hands back to your knees as you lower your head.
- Repeat 4 times.

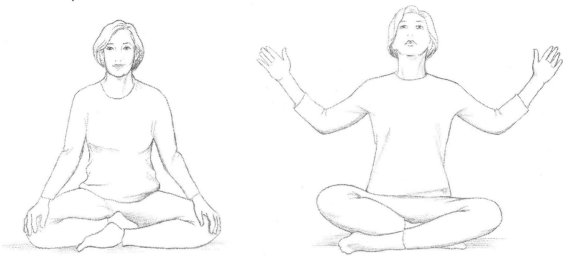

4. Rest your hands on your knees and take 10 breaths.

- Inhale for 2 counts. Hold for 3 seconds.
- Exhale free.
- With each breath, increase your inhale up to 5 counts and hold for 3 seconds after each inhale.
- Keep your exhale free.
- Repeat this series 2 times.
- Breathe freely for 10 breaths.

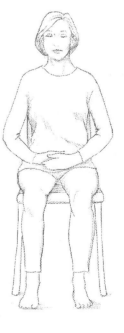

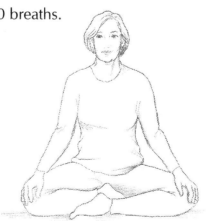

Using Your Breath Differently

The last chapter focused on breath awareness. Once you master the basics, you may want to venture into additional ways to utilize your breath to enhance the goals of your *asana* practice. Depending on whether you want to energize, balance or relax, you can adjust your breathing pattern to get the effect you wish. These techniques involve varying the length of your breath and holding it after inhale or exhale. Only attempt these variations after you've done the practices in this chapter many times.

For greater relaxation, make your exhale longer than your inhale or hold your breath briefly after exhale. We usually pause one to two seconds after each inhale and each exhale. Retaining the breath longer than two seconds is considered a hold. Initially try holding the breath one second longer than the pause. Be observant of the effect. Then you can add a second progressively up to the count of 5.

To increase your energy, hold your breath after inhale. Follow the steps outlined above.

For balancing, keep your inhale and exhale the same length and only pause for one or two seconds after each. Do not hold either your inhale or exhale longer.

Several precautions:

- The more you control the breath, the more important it is to observe the effects.
- If retaining the breath reduces the duration of your next inhale or exhale, you must discontinue this practice.
- Never hold the breath more than a count of five without the guidance of a teacher.
- If you notice tension or tightness in your chest when holding after inhale or after you start moving, discontinue this practice.

If you'd like to learn more about breath ratios, check out the resources list at the back of this book.

You Can Take It With You

The practices and principles that you've learned in this chapter, while intended for your home practice, do not need to be confined only to your mat at home. You can take them with you into the rest of your life. When you're waiting for the water to boil for tea, test your balance by doing the posture where you stand on one foot. When you're in the car stuck in traffic, use your yoga breathing instead of blowing off steam. The same holds true when you're in a long line at the supermarket: Deepen and elongate your breath to stay calm.

You might also find words or phrases that are soothing and calming for you and recite them when you need them. Here are a couple of quieting meditations that I've created. Use these as a springboard and try crafting your own set of phrases that are meaningful to you.

Breathing deep, breathing slow
Letting peace and quiet flow.
Feeling calm, feeling free
Coming home to me.

Breathing in, stillness flows
Breathing out, tension goes.
From head to toe
I am calm, I am relaxed, I am free.

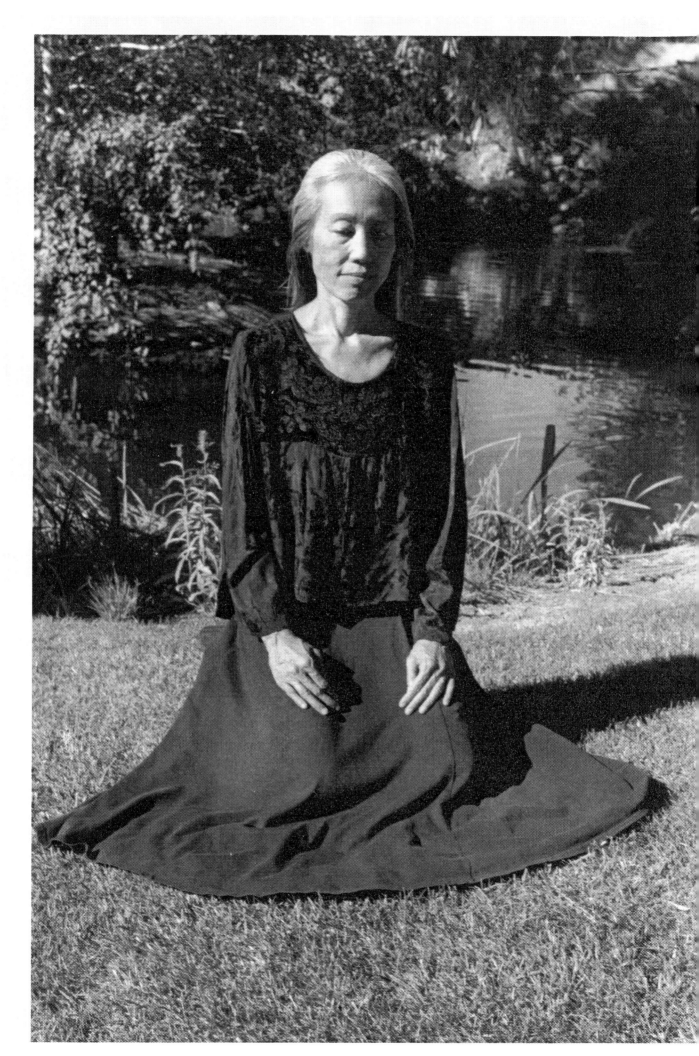

5

Meditation

You can't take your eyes off the sunset. Clouds streak across the horizon as oranges and reds shift into deep purples and pinks. Each time you blink a new formation of clouds and colors appears. You are mesmerized by the majesty of the scene before you. The phone rings. You hear a noise in the background but you don't move. You wonder, where is that coming from? It seems miles away.

Another day, you're curled up on the sofa absorbed in a novel. You can't put the book down. You don't even know where you are. The only thing real to you is the story you're reading.

Your friend, a painter, is having a similar experience in her studio. Totally immersed in her work, she doesn't know what day it is. Time flies by. She is in a state of "flow" where she is completely absorbed in pursuit of her passion.

Experiences like these take us beyond the mind, to a different realm of consciousness. You are so present, so immersed in what you're doing that you actually lose touch with everyday reality.

Are you meditating? You are certainly doing a form of meditation. And if you've had these types of experiences, you are probably a good candidate to learn the formal practice of meditation, because you've been able to detach from your surroundings and "lose" yourself in the moment.

A sitting practice of meditation takes us beyond the mind as well, so that we can experience our essential nature. The mind presents the biggest obstacle standing between awareness and our true selves. If we can move beyond our chattering minds, then we have the opportunity to discover who we truly are at our core. This is not an easy task but one that can bring lasting rewards—now and in the years ahead.

"I was introduced to meditation practice about 20 years ago, at a time in my life when I was beginning to do some self-exploration, and the path somehow led me into aikido. After six months of training, my instructor invited me to attend a class on Friday evenings that would help my aikido practice progress much more quickly. There I received my first instruction in sitting meditation. I had no idea what meditation was about, so I just did what I was told. It was difficult in the beginning, but for some reason, I persevered. As my body and mind became more relaxed over the next few years, I found myself making meditation practice an increasingly greater part of my life.

"After 20 years, I still feel like a beginner in this practice, but it has opened possibilities in my life I would not have thought possible. I found an inner strength that I did not know I had and feel more 'at home' with myself. This practice takes me to a place of kindness and strength, a refuge in times of difficulty . . . to a place of patience and wisdom, a space from which to observe the mysteries of the creation process."

—Edwina Chang, 58 (shown in chapter photo)

Why Meditate?

Many people find that as they get older, they tend to turn inward and become more reflective. As your *asana* practice develops, you may feel a tendency to go deeper as well. Meditation can add a gratifying dimension to your practice and to your life at this stage.

I can give you many reasons to meditate that have been proven by research. Studies have shown, for example, that meditation lowers heart rate, blood pressure and stress. It also increases creativity, improves your ability to focus, and enhances your perception and memory. And of course, it fosters your ability to relax.

These facts may be enough to motivate you, but most

people need a more personal incentive to begin. Here are some of the reasons I've heard that prompt people to meditate:

- To get in touch with their inner voice
- To keep their intuition and senses sharp
- To experience a sense of personal discovery
- To access inner guidance

There is no one right way to meditate. Many different approaches to meditation and many different techniques exist, each with its own language. The aim of most basic meditation techniques is similar: to relax the body, quiet the mind and cultivate mindful awareness of the present moment. In this chapter, I'm going to discuss yoga meditation as approached by T.K.V. Desikachar.

A meditation practice is very personal and ideally, you have a competent teacher to guide you in setting up a practice just for you. Since this may not be possible for you, I'm going to suggest ways to get started on your own.

You can also gain support by finding a meditation group in your town or neighborhood. If your yoga studio doesn't offer meditation, look for other possibilities that suit you nearby. It's helpful to have some guidance when you are beginning, and as you progress, you'll appreciate having the encouragement of a group. Meditating with a group creates a different kind of energy from meditating alone. Try both. Many people meditate on their own at home everyday and once or twice a week like to sit in a group or occasionally go on a group retreat. Once you have established your own meditation practice, you'll discover what combination works best for you.

Practical Questions about Meditation

Books on meditation abound. Reading about it can give you somewhat of an intellectual grounding, but you'll understand meditation best when you experience it on a visceral level. Here are the answers to some practical questions you may have in relation to meditation.

What is the Best Time of Day to Meditate?

The morning is probably the best time to meditate, for all of the same reasons that I discussed earlier on establishing your *asana* practice: you're fresh, there are fewer interruptions and you can begin your day feeling centered and grounded.

People who are avid meditators often like to practice more than once a day. Some like to add another meditation practice in late afternoon, before dinner or before bed. Practicing before breakfast and then again later in the day establishes a nice rhythm to your day.

How can I Integrate My Meditation Practice with My *Asana* and Breathing Practice?

In the classical yoga tradition, *asana* practice was considered preparation for a seated meditation, because *asana* practice generates flexibility, which, in turn, makes it easier to sit without tiring or pain. This principle holds true today.

If you don't have time to do your full asana practice before you meditate, then do something shorter, such as the ten-minute practice in the last chapter. You can also meditate sitting on a chair, which is less stressful on your body than sitting on the floor on a cushion.

That said, there are also advantages to meditating before doing your *asana* practice, especially in the morning. If you roll out of bed and meditate, you can bring a quieter, less distracted quality of mind to your sitting, which may help you go deeper.

How Long is Long Enough to Meditate?

As with your *asana* practice, it's a good idea to start with a shorter practice and build on it than to begin with a long practice and get discouraged, because you can't sit for the whole time you've allotted. You can start sitting for five or ten minutes and see how that goes. Try that for a week or two, and then begin adding time, if you want to.

You can also stay with a shorter meditation. If you're doing an asana practice that lasts 30–40 minutes, a ten-minute meditation may feel like enough. You can experiment with this over time and see what length of meditation practice is satisfying for you and what blends in with the rest of your day. Like your *asana* practice, your mediation practice should be something that you look forward to, not a heavy "should" that hangs around your neck.

Do I need a Particular Focus?

The guiding principle—that you need a specific focus for your meditation—applies to most forms of meditation. This can be a concrete object, your breath, a meaningful word or passage, or a question of inquiry. What's most important is that the object has significance or interest for you.

How Important is the Position I Sit In?

You don't need to sit in a particular position to meditate. The quality of your meditation will not be affected in any way if you sit on a chair or in another seated position on the floor. Your sitting *will* be affected by discomfort, however, so select a position that is comfortable for you.

Try one of the positions shown here or a seated position of your own choosing that works for you. The three most common positions are:

- Seated on the floor in a crossed-legged position. If you choose to sit this way, it is important to have your knees level with or below your hips. If you are having difficulty maintaining an erect spine while sitting cross-legged, raise your hips by sitting on the edge of a cushion, bolster, or rolled blanket. For additional support, place rolled blankets or bolsters under your knees.

- Seated on your heels with a pillow under your hips or resting on a meditation stool.

- Seated upright in a chair. The chair should be firm, your back straight, and your feet flat on the floor or supported with a book or cushion under them.

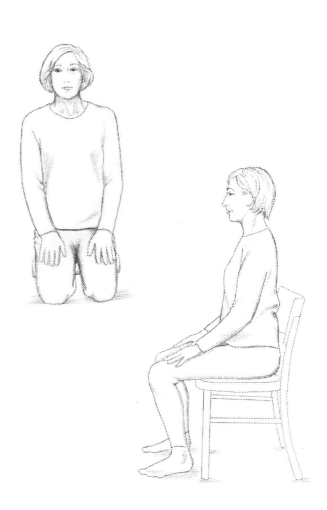

"My experience with chronic pain and fatigue, which began in 1986, has been one of loss and self-reinvention. Finally diagnosed with fibromyalgia in 1995, I discovered some of the most useful healing practices involve accessing the universal energy the Chinese call chi.

"For about six years I studied Chi Kung. Although I could not do all the forms, Chi Kung greatly enhanced my range of motion and flexibility, and the meditative aspect provided another avenue for spiritual healing. But when my teachers moved away from Santa Fe, my practice began to dwindle.

"By chance, I met a yoga teacher who offered a class for people in mid-life and older, who was willing to consider my physical limitations—albeit fewer than before I discovered Chi Kung. Again I found I could improve flexibility and range of motion, strengthen bone and muscle, balance mood, and release stress and anxiety. I had to experiment to determine which poses triggered pain, whether immediately or with delayed onset.

"Through trial and error and working individually with my teacher, I now have a repertoire of poses that when approached gently and with focus have produced holistic results similar to what I was achieving with Chi Kung. By not holding the poses for too long, or pushing too far, I can create some of the more flowing motion I had found so enjoyable and beneficial, and tap into the same life force.

"Today I practice yoga once a week with my group. At home, I practice a mixture of Chi Kung and yoga. The commonality of breath and intention in moving the body and settling the mind make these two practices highly complimentary. I feel blessed that both these paths have led to compassionate healing as well as prevention."

—Rosemary Thompson, 59

What if I Don't Feel Drawn to Meditation?

Not everyone is drawn to a seated meditation practice. If you are one of these people, it's nothing to be concerned about. If you become interested in it at some later date, you can pursue it then. Or you may continue to feel that your *asana* and breathing practice is enough. And that's fine too. Whatever you choose to do, don't criticize yourself for not wanting to meditate. Just accept that this is how you feel now.

What's the Best Way to Get Started?

Try one or all three of the following as an introduction to seated meditation. If, after this trial sitting, you feel pulled toward meditation and want to go deeper, then follow the detailed steps outlined in the next section of this chapter.

- Sit quietly for ten minutes. Close the door, turn off the ringer on your phone, and just sit. Observe your thoughts as they come and go. Try not to judge yourself, simply notice where your mind goes. This experiment will give you some idea of the degree to which your mind is restless and agitated.

- Observe your breath. Direct all your attention to your inhale and exhale. You can even say, "inhale" as you inhale and "exhale" as you exhale. When you mind starts to wander, as it invariably will, notice where it goes—again without judging yourself—and gently bring it back to your breath. Sit for ten minutes focusing on your breath.

- Visualize loving kindness. As you sit and breathe, focus on your heart center and imagine thoughts of loving, caring and nurturing emanating from it. Direct those thoughts to someone whom you know who is ill or who needs extra nurturing. If you need such caring yourself, then visualize yourself bathed in warmth and kindness. Sit for ten minutes.

Is There a Special Way to Prepare for Meditation?

Some people just sit down and begin. To have a smoother transition from your everyday life to your sitting, however, you can do some gentle movement, such as the meditative practice in the last chapter. You can also try breathing consciously or select a reading of a spiritual nature to establish the tone for your meditation practice. You may also want to set an intention before you begin. Do this by selecting an issue that you want to explore through your meditation, such as your focus, attention or a particular inquiry.

The Meditation Itself

It is very difficult to describe in words what actually happens when you meditate. You will truly understand it when you experience it yourself. The following guidelines will help you get started.

Yoga meditation involves three steps:

1. Choosing an Object.

Select an object that is meaningful for you that will help you turn inward and focus your mind. In the beginning it's useful to use an external object, because it is concrete and tangible and gives you a clear focusing point.

You can choose a physical object, like the mountains or a stream, or the photograph of someone you respect or love, such as your teacher or guru, who embodies qualities that you would like to have, or something with an existing religious or spiritual connection. You can also use a symbolic image, like a color or a pleasing sound. Your breath can also serve as the object.

T.K.V. Desikachar advises, "...start with something to which you can relate. In yoga it is said that you must begin where you are and with what you like.... What is important is that the chosen object does not cause you any problems or hinder you from focusing your mind." For example, a Muslim in India would have difficulty meditating on the word OM because that is the holy sound of the Hindu culture, just as a Jewish person would struggle with meditating on a cross.

Select an object that is imbued with positive qualities for you, rather than one with a negative charge. You may need to experiment with several different objects until you find one that resonates with you.

2. Linking to an Object or Question

After you have chosen the object, connect with it. You can do this in several ways. Say you have selected the mountains as your object, because they represent stability, constancy, and strength, qualities that you'd like to possess. In linking with them, you concentrate on these qualities as a way to make them a part of your life.

You can also connect with the object by asking for guidance or clarity about key questions or immediate concerns in your life. You might ask: What is my purpose or role in life? Who am I? What does my future hold? Connecting with your object, through asking a question, enables you to clear your mind and reflect on the issues you have raised— without the usual distractions that accompany daily life.

3. Meditating on the Object

Experience the object in whatever way you can. Absorb it into your being. Let go of analyzing and thinking, and merge with it. If you've ever experienced "flow," that intense concentration when you're writing or painting and completely lose sense of time and place, you've had a taste of the attentiveness and focus that meditation creates.

Complete your meditation by using one of the same transitional activities you began with: Do some gentle movements or conscious breathing, study a reading that's meaningful to you, or recite aloud a favorite poem or passage. End with an expression of gratitude to help draw your sitting experience into your daily life. Then, moving slowly and deliberately, shift into the rest of your day.

Attitudes Toward Sitting

Certain attitudes will help you have a positive experience sitting. Of course, it is important that you come to meditation with the same nonjudgmental and uncompetitive mind-set that you bring to your *asana* practice. Here are few other attitudes that will enhance your sitting practice:

- *Let go.* When you have distracting thoughts or emotions while you're sitting, notice what they are and let them go by redirecting your mind back to your object. Avoid giving them your attention or criticizing yourself for having them. Everyone experiences them. Simply observe them and return to your intention. If you feel these thoughts are important, write them down and return to your practice.

- *Accept whatever arises.* You don't know what will come up when you meditate. That's the beauty of the unknown. Acknowledge whatever feelings, thoughts, or emotions occur—be they good, bad or indifferent. They are all part of you and your experiences. When you are feeling them, be assured that you are not alone. Many others have had the same emotions.

- *Set reasonable expectations.* Come to sitting with an open mind and an open heart. Meditation is a process that deepens over time. See what happens. Results differ from day to day. Consistent practice will have an effect.

- *Take your time.* Don't rush. While you are sitting, imagine that you have nothing else to do and nowhere to go. Let your meditation evolve at its own pace and in its own time. Flow with it wherever it takes you.

Meditation Cultivates Awareness

Just as we practice yoga on the mat and "off the mat," so heightened awareness can also extend beyond the formal practice, and into the rest of your life. Walk slowly and consciously. Bring focus and one-pointedness to any activity you do. Even washing the dishes can be a meditation if done with single-mindedness and concentration. Rather than multi-tasking, do one thing at a time and give that activity your complete attention. This will help you feel more focused and less scattered, and you'll actually get more done than if you do several things once.

Take time each day to notice and appreciate your surroundings. You may walk past the same oak tree every day and not see it. Really look at it the next time you go by.

Gaze into the eyes of someone you love and truly see him or her, as though you've just returned from a long trip. Think about what you cherish about your partner, friend or grandchild and then connect with those feelings.

As you continue practicing meditation and bring the qualities of awareness and consciousness more frequently into your life, you'll see positive changes in the quality of your own life and a new richness in your relationships.

6

Living Yoga

For many years, I attended yoga class regularly. I loved coming to class. I always felt relaxed and clear after I left, but I had no desire to practice at home or to delve any deeper into the study of yoga. When I took my teacher training, I learned that the key to being an effective teacher lay in having your own regular personal practice. That was my goal, so I began practicing at home. It was that simple. And once I started practicing on my own, I was captivated. I couldn't start my day *without* my yoga practice. I needed it. If I missed a day, the morning started a little shaky. I felt off-center all day and was much more reactive to people and situations that arose in the course of the day.

During my teacher training, the director often made references to classical yoga philosophy, especially to the *Yoga Sutra*. It is believed that the *Yoga Sutra* dates from between the fourth century BCE and the fourth century CE. The sage Patanjali compiled the existing yoga knowledge into four books of aphorisms that were subsequently passed down orally from teacher to student. Our word *suture* comes from *sutra*, which links the teacher, the teaching and the student. The books offer insights into psychological, philosophical and spiritual questions.

The director's references to the *Sutras* piqued my curiosity, but I had no avenue for exploring them further. When I moved to Santa Fe, I welcomed the opportunity to join a weekly *Sutra* study group.

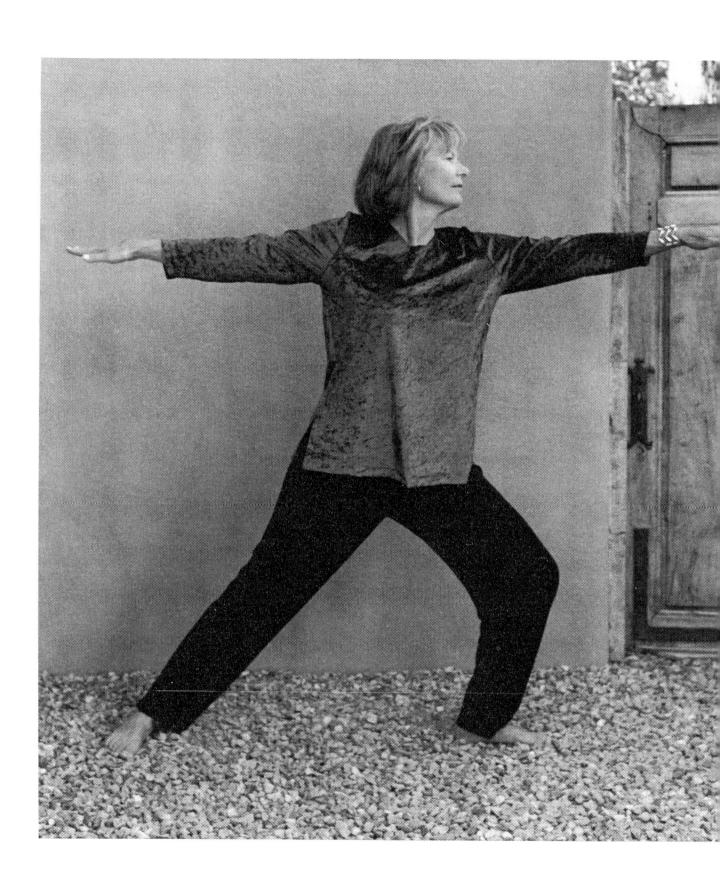

Studying the *Sutras* have added enormous depth to my practice and study of yoga and have helped integrate yoga into the rest of my life. There are so many lessons for living consciously and thoughtfully. These concepts are just as relevant today as they were when they were written thousands of years ago.

And they are particularly pertinent to us as we age. Of course, we want to be strong and flexible—that's one of the reasons we practice. But rather than only being concerned about the physical form of our postures, at this stage of our lives we want to go deeper: to delve beneath the surface and use yoga to get to know ourselves in a more fundamental, spiritual way.

We've seen how conscious breathing and meditation can bring our practices to a different level. To deepen your practice even further and broaden it, I want to introduce some concepts from the *Yoga Sutras*. I've chosen the ones that have been most meaningful for me. When you study classical yoga philosophy on your own, you may find other concepts that are more personally relevant to you, but for now, start with these. Think about them, reflect on the questions posed, and stay open to how they might give you a different perspective on your own life.

Rather than quoting the entire aphorism, I have selected key concepts and words. This is one of the few parts of the book in which I'm using Sanskrit because I believe it adds a texture to the definition, and as you become more involved in yoga and begin building a support system, you may feel more comfortable and knowledgeable when you hear these words used.

Living Your Yoga

It's All Connected

According to ancient teachings that predate the *Yoga Sutra*, the human system is structured from the gross to the subtle, from the more external to the more internal. The layers, called **mayas** (also referred to as **koshas** or **maya koshas**) in Sanskrit, consist of:

- The physical level, which is supported by doing yoga postures
- The energetic level associated with breathing
- The mental level maintained by education and learning
- A deeper, innate intelligence, including personality and inborn as well as conditioned tendencies
- The subtlest level, that of emotions, joy and devotion.

The *mayas* are not hierarchical; they all influence and interact with each other. For example, we know that the breath reflects the state of the mind and can calm it. We also know that doing yoga postures—a physical act—influences the mind and the emotions. Certain *mayas* dominate at certain times. None of these is negative, but we need to keep them in balance. Ideally, we want to function from our deepest intelligence with the mind being a useful tool.

Questions to think about:

- At what level do you usually respond?
- In what ways to do you notice one level affecting the others? For example, how do you feel physically, energetically, and emotionally after doing a strong *asana* practice?
- When you feel mentally dull, how are your other levels affected?
- On the other hand, when you feel content, what do you notice about the other levels?

I notice, for example, that if I don't get enough sleep, all parts of my system are affected: I feel dull mentally and lack physical energy. I feel disheartened about aspects of my life that usually don't disturb me, and even facets of my life that make me happy on a day when I'm rested seem lackluster when I don't get enough sleep.

I introduce the *mayas* to show the interrelatedness of the following concepts. In the *Yoga Sutra*, some of these ideas pertain to the physical practice of yoga, but they can also be interpreted on a broader, psychological level. When applied to living situations, they can serve as a tool for increasing your self-awareness.

"Psychoanalyst C.G. Jung believed that the mellowing of the soul is compensation for the deterioration of the body. For me, yoga supports, nurtures and sustains both body and soul. The integration of breath and movement slows and calms me down. I feel more centered, focused and present in the moment as I seek to restore the natural rhythm of my body. The various poses stretch, lengthen and strengthen my body and I particularly like savasana, the corpse pose at the end of each session, when I am at one with eternity. I appreciate being in a class designed for people in midlife where the rhythm and pace are just right and I don't feel rushed or inadequate.

"As I enter my early 60's I am seeking deeper meanings, and my attention turns more inward, to the whisperings of the inner voice and the soul's calling. Yoga is a helpful companion on my journey inward. I know the best years are still to come."

—Gabrilla Hoeglund, 61 (shown on page 140)

Stability/Ease

In an *asana* practice, we try to balance firmness and stability with comfort and ease. In Sanskrit these opposing but complementary qualities are called **sthira** and **sukha.** We strive for relaxation in a posture but we don't want to become so laid back that we doze off. On the other hand, we also want strength but not to the point of strain. It is a delicate balance. According to T.K.V. Desikachar, "It is attention without tension, loosening-up without slackness."

The first step in achieving this sense of equilibrium is an awareness that we're not in balance: We notice that we're too lax or trying too hard. Then we adjust our practice so that we don't veer too far in one direction. An intention to observe these qualities may lead to a greater sense of balance between them. Likewise, once *sthira* and *sukha* are in balance in a particular practice, we're better able to observe ourselves. Out of this observation comes a sense of discovery.

As we learn to observe and balance *sthira* and *sukha* as an integral part of practice, these qualities affect the rest of our lives. They teach us how to be steady and stable in a world that's always changing. We learn to cope with opposites, such as pleasure and pain, and success and failure, without being overwhelmed or overpowered by an extreme. Over time, the balance and stability we gain from our practice helps us cope with change by becoming less attached to the outcome.

How these qualities play out in your own life can be revealing. Think about these questions:

- How adaptable are you to new situations?
- When do you feel overpowered or overwhelmed?
- What is your response to these situations?
- In your relationships, do you take a rigid stance or are you firm but giving?
- In your beliefs, how open are you to new ideas?
- In challenging situations, are you always serious or can you use humor to lighten things up?

After you've considered these questions, think about what patterns exist between the balance of *sthira* and *sukha* in your *asana* practice and in your daily behavior. The connections may surprise you.

For myself, I notice that when I consciously balance *sthira* and *sukha* in my yoga practice, I am much more even-tempered in my life. If I don't give these two qualities enough attention or they are out of balance, I am much more reactive and less considerate in my relationships with other people.

Our Attitudes to Others and to Ourselves

The attitudes we have toward other people are called **yamas** in Sanskrit. These include how we interact with and relate to others and the environment, and our approach to people. Most of these are self-explanatory. The *yamas* are:

- Nonviolence or *ahimsa*
- Truthfulness or *satya*
- Not coveting what belongs to others or *asteya*
- Responsible behavior in moving toward the truth is known as *brahmacarya*. In the past this term was associated with abstinence, particularly to the stage of life of the student, but today it has the broader meaning of moving toward and understanding what's essential in life.
- Not taking more than is necessary or appropriate in a given situation is called *aparigraha* in Sanskrit.

The attitudes we adopt toward ourselves are called **niyamas** in Sanskrit. These are much more intimate and personal than the *yamas,* as they only include our attitudes to ourselves, not to other people. They are:

- Cleanliness or *sauca*: cleanliness in your body, both internally and externally, and in your surroundings
- Contentment or *santosa*: being comfortable with what we have and what we don't have, as well as accepting what happens to us
- A process of removing impurities called *tapas* (see below)
- Self-observation, known as *svadhyaya* (see below)
- To act without being attached to the fruits of your actions is called *ishvarapranidhana* (see below)

Together, the *yamas* and *niyamas* provide attitudes and behaviors to live by. Practicing yoga can make us more aware of these attitudes and help us change them in a desired direction. In fact, the degree to which we practice the *yamas* and *niyamas* can serve as a barometer for the effectiveness of our yoga practice. When we reflect on them, they can show us how to find happiness internally, how to live consciously and thoughtfully in the world, and how to develop and maintain healthy relationships.

Here is a practical way to give these principles relevance in your daily life. I'll use contentment as an example, but the following 3 steps can be applied with variations to each of the attitudes above.

1. Notice when you're not feeling content.
2. Observe what form your discontent takes. It could be in the form of entitlement, trying too hard, feeling dissatisfied or impatient, or having unreasonable expectations.
3. Decide what you're going to do about it. You have several choices:
   • Live with it consciously and see what happens.
   • Try to understand why this has occurred or what's behind it.
   • Introduce a foil for it, just as we do a counterpose in yoga practice. Following a backbend, for example, we neutralize the effects of stretching backwards by doing a forward bend to balance ourselves. To counteract discontent, you might actively cultivate an attitude of gratitude.

"Yoga has helped me achieve growing clarity and acceptance. My study of the Yoga Sutra, novice that I am, has given me a model for understanding the human system and for living with self-acceptance, compassion and faith.

"My yoga teacher has had the greatest influence in guiding me from a vision of yoga focused on asana to one in which our goal is moving deeper. Not more poses—deeper. Going within, not staying on the surface.

"Self-acceptance has been one of the most important areas in which I have had to grow. Going through menopause, I felt a sense a shame about growing older. The physical changes of age became very visible to me. As a yoga teacher, I had felt I needed to present myself in a certain way—thin, youthful, strong, ever flexible, master of all kinds of poses. Through examining those images that our culture presents and we internalize, I have gained a sense of freedom in letting them go.

"Today, I like my post-menopausal self, a woman of 56. My practice is about what I need, not what I think I should do to meet someone's image of a yoga teacher. While asana is part of my practice and teaching, it takes place within the larger frame of yoga. My goal is to walk a path in which I might somehow bring some greater peace and healing into the small part of the world through which I pass. For that yoga is my guide."

—Elizabeth Terry, 56

Yoga of Action

The last three **yamas** are also part of what is known as **kriya yoga** or the yoga of action. Because these qualities provide such important insights into our behavior and motivation, I want to give them a fuller explanation.

- Removing impurities, called **tapas**, is a way to keep healthy mentally, physically, emotionally, and spiritually. It involves a process of inner cleansing in order to eliminate what we don't need. We "burn up" old ways of doing things to keep us fresh. This brings more attention to our behavior. It is any action that you intentionally do differently.

For example, if you always do your yoga practice at 8 a.m. in the same room and do the postures in the same order, after awhile, the practice can become mechanical and stale. This is the time to introduce a *tapas*, something different to revitalize you. You might try practicing at 5 p.m. or in a different room of the house. Or you might keep the hour and the room the same but add a new awareness, such as attentiveness to "the pause" in your practice. Any of these changes will shake up things for you. They may cause some discomfort initially but eventually, they'll bring more awareness to your practice, and more pleasure.

Tapas can also be applied to areas outside of your yoga practice. You can bring it into your relationships. Sit in your husband's "seat" at the dinner table and see what happens. If you always voice your dissatisfaction in the form of a complaint, try using humor instead.

Think about the ways you can add your own unique *tapas* to your personal practice, to your daily life and to your relationships.

- Self-observation, known as **svadhyaya,** originated as a way to study the sacred Vedic texts and use them for self-understanding. It also includes studying and observing yourself through action. One way to observe yourself is to sit back at the end of the day and reflect on your actions or write in a journal. But *svadhyaya* is more than that: it is being attentive *while things are happening.* Say you do the *tapas* suggested above of sitting in your husband's seat at dinner. The next step would be to observe yourself: Are you anxious about initiating this change? How do you feel actually sitting there? What is his response? How do you respond to him? Through observation at the time you will know the effect of the *tapas*.

Ideally, self-observation occurs naturally all the time, but the reality is, without some intention, this doesn't happen. The following questions may help you become more aware of the times when you observe yourself and in what situations you need more attentiveness:

- In general, how much awareness do you usually have?
- In which situations are you routinely observant of yourself?
- What kinds of situations or emotions prevent you from being observant?
- What can you do to increase your self-observational skills?

Your ability to observe yourself will improve the more you do it and the more you tune in to how you're feeling at the moment. These observations, however, should be made without judgments. You simply observe; you do not criticize yourself for *what* you're observing. For most people, this requires a conscious effort and is the most difficult part of *svadhyaya*.

- Acting without becoming attached to the fruits of your action is called **ishvarapranidhana**. In some contexts, this means surrendering to a Higher Power but it also has the broader meaning of letting go or taking an action with an attitude of openness to the result. You have no expectations of how a situation will turn out or what the other person will do. You go in receptive to whatever may happen.

One of the benefits of this kind of surrendering is that it brings about a sense of humility. You have an awareness that you're not in control of the outcome but you move forward anyway, not knowing the consequences of your actions and being open to whatever that may be.

A way to achieve this is to think of your action as an offering. When you give an offering, it is done graciously and selflessly with no concern for "What's in it for me?" or "What am I going to get back?" You simply act and see what happens.

The three parts of *kriya* yoga work together: Doing *tapas* provokes you out of your comfort zone. *Svadhyaya* allows you to observe yourself in a new or unusual context. *Ishvarapranidhana* enables you to be open to whatever the consequences may be of this new situation.

Incorrect Understanding

When we see situations and behavior of others and ourselves clearly, we're more likely to act with clarity and lucidity. Unfortunately, this is not always the case. Often we operate from incorrect knowledge, false understanding, or clouded perceptions. This is called **avidya** in Sanskrit and is a major source of difficulty in our relationships with others and with ourselves. *Avidya* is the inability to distinguish between:

- What's me and what's not me
- What's permanent and what's changing
- What's painful and what's pleasant
- What's pure and what's impure

There are four ways that *avidya* can be experienced:

1. Association/identification, known as **asmita** in Sanskrit (in Western terms, the functioning of the ego)

This occurs when you have either too much ego ("I am terrific" or "I am always right") or too little. For example, perhaps you don't distinguish between what you do and who you are. I went through a period when I over-identified as a writer to the point that when my workload was down, I felt as though I had little worth as a person. Too much of my ego was wrapped up in my writing. This can also occur if you over-identify with your children's accomplishments. Think of the parent of a child in Little League who berates his son for striking out or pushes him beyond his capabilities just so the parent can boast about his talented offspring.

2. Excessive attachment or desire, known as ***raga.***

This is associated with pleasure seeking that gets out of hand. Yes, you can have too much of a good thing. Think about when your daughter was madly in love: her excessive and obsessive connection prevented her from seeing her boyfriend realistically. *Raga* frequently occurs around food. Who can eat one piece of chocolate or one potato chip? Of course, one piece is good but it's not nearly enough: you *must* eat more. When you hear yourself say, "I want ..." perk up and pay attention. Then sit back and ask yourself:

- Do I really need this?
- What will it mean if I have it?
- What can I do to counteract the desire?

This is the time to bring in something to thwart your desire, just as I discussed cultivating gratitude when you're feeling discontent earlier in this chapter. In the case of wanting more chocolate or chips, you consciously do something to re-direct your desire and divert your attention, such as eating a piece of fruit or taking a walk. Also, imagining the negative consequences of following through on your impulse (extra pounds on the hips) can act as a deterrent.

3. Unreasonable dislike or aversion, know as ***dvesha.***

Dvesha in some ways is the opposite of *raga.* You have a negative experience in the past and because you don't want to repeat it, you automatically reject the people or setting surrounding the experience, assuming that it will be negative again.

If you find yourself unusually negative and rejecting, consider:

- Where is this negativity coming from?
- Am I blaming others for a past hurt?
- Is my reaction over the top? If so, what might be causing it?
- Am I overreacting to a current situation because of something that happened in the past?

4. Generalized fear or anxiety, known as ***abhinevesha.***

This is an existential anxiety or apprehension with regard to the unknown and includes fear of death. This type of anxiety is part of life. Everyone experiences this, but some people feel it more strongly and more frequently than others. It expresses itself in the following ways:

- Feeling a lack of confidence
- Being afraid of being judged by others
- Doubting yourself
- Having anxiety about losing what you have
- Feeling fearful of growing older

How do we know that we're experiencing clouded perceptions or incorrect knowledge? We suffer. That's the bad news. The good news is that we can do something about these mistaken perceptions, because they are all self-induced. Therefore, changing them is under our control.

"The least safe place for me on the planet has always been inside my own body. For years I have carried the memory of trauma with me, in the tension of my shoulders, in my shallow, panicked breathing, in the wall of fat I've hidden behind, in my inability to find balance, either physical or mental.

"Now, after years of hard work in therapy, after most of the psychological healing has happened, I've found in yoga a way to be in my body without fear. Just now, at 60, I am learning how to breathe. In this class I'm learning to relax and to fall asleep. I am learning to pay attention to how I feel when I eat. I'm not afraid that someone will ridicule my body because we are all older women, and there is no competition among us. I am not afraid to make mistakes because this yoga class is utterly forgiving and I don't have to be perfect to avoid being attacked. Slowly, week by week, I am getting my body back. To quote a meditation we share in class sometimes, I feel that I am coming home to me."

— Carol Eastes, 60

Suffering

Everyone from the Buddha to pop authors has acknowledged that life contains suffering. In yogic philosophy, the Sanskrit word **duhkha** covers pain of all sorts, including misery and discomfort of an emotional nature. You don't have to be in a crisis to experience *duhkha*. You know you're in *duhkha* when you experience one of the following:

- Feeling conflicted or restricted
- Wanting to be someplace else
- Feeling a tinge of dis - ease
- Yearning to turn the clock back to undo an action or occurrence

Duhkha often results when you act from *avidya*. You may not realize it at the time. You only feel the pain, but if you look closer, you may realize that you're coping with the emotions of selfishness, desire, hate or fear.

Duhkha is also a sign. It's a way of telling you that you need to practice on a more regular basis or deepen your existing practice. For some people, in fact, practice consists only of *duhkha* management. This is fine, but your practice also has the potential to be much more.

Duhkha can be anticipated and avoided. Practicing on a regular basis, even when things are going well, can help deter *duhkha*. Practice gives us distance so we can anticipate when *duhkha* is coming. Then, we don't have to expend energy coping with the consequences.

Everything is Real. Everything Changes.

One way to reduce *duhkha* is to incorporate this thought into your life: Everything is real but everything changes. This concept, **sat vada, parinama vada** in Sanskrit, can be explored on many levels: mental, physical, emotional and spiritual.

Consider the physical level. Last week when you did tree pose in yoga class, you had no problem balancing on one leg. Today you feel shaky and can barely lift one foot off the floor without losing your balance. Each day you wake up feeling differently. Maybe you didn't sleep well last night or you heard some distressing news this morning before class. All these things influence your abilities in your yoga practice.

This concept has been most helpful to me when I'm coping with personal problems or emotional difficulties. By the time we reach midlife, we've all been through something: a health problem of our own, angst with a child, a death or a divorce. This concept reminds me that what I'm going through is real, but that it will change. It gives me a perspective on the problem. Say you're going through the very early stages of grieving following the death of a loved one. Your feelings are intense; you think you're never going to feel better. If you can step back and realize that "what I'm feeling is real but it will change," you can gain some distance from the difficulty and put it into perspective. It's realizing that this, too, will pass.

Taking Yoga Home

I began this book by saying that yoga is a homecoming, a coming home to ourselves. All these concepts have one thing in common: They lead us home. They are ways to get to know ourselves better, to strip away the artifacts and to get in touch with our inner voices. Then, we can act and respond from our core, authentic selves rather than being swayed by the latest fad that breezes in.

Studying yoga—examining concepts from classical yoga philosophy in some combination with doing a practice of postures, breathing and meditation—is a lifelong process. Take your time. Move at your own pace. Follow your own path. Seek a teacher when you need guidance. Attend classes when you need additional support and stimulation.

Yoga can be your companion in the years ahead as you navigate the decades to come. Be reassured that you are not alone. You have a long, solid tradition behind you with a set of practices and principles that can help you face whatever lies ahead. Take what you need from these and make it your own. Create a personal practice that honors your past, embraces who you are today, and prepares you for the future.

Welcome home!

Resources

Desikachar, T.K.V. *The Heart of Yoga: Developing a Personal Practice.* Rochester (VT): Inner Traditions International; 1995.

Desikachar, T.K.V. *Reflections on Yoga Sutra-s of Patanjali.* Chennai: Krishnamacharya Yoga Mandiram; 1987. To order, contact www.kym.org

Bachman, Nicolai. *The Language of Yoga.* Boulder (CO): Sounds True; 2005.

Bouanchaud, Bernard. *The Essence of Yoga: Reflections on the Yoga Sutras of Patanjali.* Portland (OR): Rudra Press; 1997.

Harvey, Paul. *Yoga for Every Body.* Pleasantville (NY): Reader's Digest Association; 2001.

Kraftsow, Gary. *Yoga for Wellness: Healing with the Timeless Teachings of Viniyoga.* New York: Penguin/Arkana; 1999.

Nelson, Sonia. *Patanjali's Yoga Sutra: A Chanting Tutorial.* Santa Fe (NM); 2002. To order, contact www.vedicchantcenter.org

Pierce, Margaret D. and Martin G. *Yoga for Your Life: A Practice Manual of Breath and Movement for Every Body.* Portland (OR): Rudra Press; 1996.

The typeface used throughout this book
is CG Omega, a true type font.

Printed in the United States
65464LVS00002B

9 780865 344990